"*Buff Dad* is a perfect book for the father who has gotten out of shape or has never been in shape and does not have time to go to the gym and spend all day there. Mike has worked with me to get me in tip-top shape. I have two young children and my time is spent with my kids or working on a movie, so when it comes to working out, I want a quick and intense workout. *Buff Dad* has the answer for dads of all ages and fitness levels. If you follow the workout plan and diet portion, you are guaranteed to be a Buff Dad."

—Morris Chestnut
actor, *The Best Man, The Brothers*

"Gaining weight during your wife's pregnancy seems crazy, unlikely, and a simple problem to overcome. But until you've gone through those beautiful nine months alongside your significant other, and then the change in your life after the birth, it's hard to describe. The idea of wanting to spend every moment with your new bundle of joy sidetracks you to the point where you can't imagine how fast the weight grabs you (fifteen pounds here). *Buff Dad* shows you how to care for your family while caring for yourself at the same time! If you don't care for your own body, you won't be around to be able to care for someone else's."

—Kevin Sizemore
actor, with roles in *Without a Trace, 24, CSI Miami, Jag*

"What a pleasant surprise *Buff Dad* was. Not only does Mike Levinson know what he's talking about, the book is actually a funny, insightful read for any dad. A great no-nonsense way to get your fitness act back together."

—James Denton
actor, *Desperate Housewives*

D0905138

BUFF DAD

The 4-Week Fitness Game Plan for Real Guys

MIKE LEVINSON, R.D.
and Michelle Ponto

Health Communications, Inc.
Deerfield Beach, Florida

www.hcibooks.com

Library of Congress Cataloging-in-Publication Data

Levinson, Mike.
    Buff dad : the 4-week fitness game plan for real guys / Mike Levinson and Michelle Ponto.
    p. cm.
    Includes bibliographical references and index.
    ISBN-13: 978-0-7573-0616-7 (trade paper)
    ISBN-10: 0-7573-0616-0 (trade paper)
    1. Reducing diets. 2. Weight loss. 3. Men—Health and hygiene. 4. Fathers—Health
and hygiene. I. Ponto, Michelle. II. Title.
    RM222.2.L444 2008
    613.2'5—dc22
                                2007048396

Publisher: Health Communications, Inc.
          3201 S.W. 15th Street
          Deerfield Beach, FL 33442-8190

Cover design by Larissa Hise Henoch
Interior design and formatting by Lawna Patterson Oldfield

This book is dedicated to my wife, Jennifer, who has stood by and supported me throughout this long journey. I could not have done this without her. I wake up each morning and thank my lucky stars for her in my life.

Also my three sons, Zach, Ben, and Josh—I could not be a buff dad without you. I love you all! Also I look forward to my other twin boys, who will be born in a few months, for allowing me to be a buff dad!

A special thanks to my agent, Linda Konner, who has believed in me and never gave up.

CONTENTS

PART I

YOU'RE AN OVERWEIGHT DAD— NOW WHAT?

CHAPTER 1

FROM FITNESS TRAINER TO FAT DAD

The Birth of the *Buff Dad* Program

To be a great champion, you must believe you are the best.
If you're not, pretend you are.

Muhammad Ali

I t's surprising how fast it happens. One day you're fit, lean, and able to race up a flight of stairs without breaking a sweat. Then suddenly you're overweight, soft in the middle, and can't see your toes when you look down.

Deep down we all know the fat fairy didn't visit us in our sleep and zap us with her love-handle–making wand. But while some of us can blame the unexpected weight gain on genetics or growing older, for many of us the reality is that something else changed in our lives: we became fathers.

Even though we had nine months to prepare, it wasn't enough for this wonderful, yet life-altering experience. I know. Five years ago, I became a father myself.

Just like the thousands of men who become first-time dads every year in North America, I was completely unaware of how the miracle of fatherhood was about to change my life. While I love my son, and his birth has brought new meaning to my life, I wasn't ready for what was about to happen to both my life and my body.

The Miracle of Fatherhood

I clearly remember the day we took my son home from the hospital and placed him in the nursery. As I watched his chest rise and fall as he slept, I suddenly realized the nursery wasn't the only thing that was different in our home. I was different, too. I was someone's dad—and it was amazing, scary, and exciting all at the same time.

As you know, fatherhood not only changes you mentally, but it also creates an entirely new dynamic in your personal life. Gone are the weekends of sleeping in, the impulsive nights out, and the freewheeling daily routine you once had. Overnight, everything shifts to accommodate someone else's schedule.

Before you know it, you realize you haven't gone for your morning run in eight months, you've eaten more baby cookies and Goldfish crackers than you care to admit, and you vaguely remember seeing your home gym somewhere behind the stroller and portable playpen. The scary thing is, you don't really care, nor do you miss your old self.

Then the inevitable happens. One morning you wake up and realize you've become the one thing you never thought you'd be: fat.

The Road to Poundage Is Paved with Calories

Working in the fitness field as a personal trainer and nutritionist for most of my adult life, I never had a problem making time to go to the gym. It was part of my daily routine and how I made my living. In my industry, I was fortunate to have worked with some of the top athletic organizations in North America, including the Chicago Bears and the Oakland Raiders.

My clients included celebrities and professional athletes such as Chris Oakley, J. T. Snow, and Sean Rooks of the NBA. I spent my days working with each of my clients on an individual basis, focusing on achieving long-term results through challenging and constantly varied workouts. And with my master's degree in sports nutrition, I was able to help them not only build muscle and lose weight in the gym, but fine-tune their eating habits. In fact, my expertise in functional training and some of my innovative fitness techniques are widely recognized in the industry.

I was also a former amateur bodybuilding champion, so I know how good my body can look and how it feels to be in shape. I spent my whole life living, breathing, and preaching good health. Never in a million years did I believe I would ever get fat.

My friends and coworkers warned me that my life would change when the baby came, but I didn't believe them. I was convinced they were using fatherhood as an excuse to let themselves go. I imagined them going home, turning on the television, pushing back the reclining chair, and eating potato chips while their child played peacefully in the baby activity center.

Up there on my child-free pedestal I swore that I would never be "that" dad. How could I? I wasn't the one who had gained 20 to 30 pounds in nine months. I was the father. Besides changing a couple of diapers and waking up for some morning feedings, how different would my life be?

It turned out the joke was on me. With the birth of my son, everything changed. Just like every other dad out there, my priorities changed. In addition to my career and the everyday chores of grocery shopping, car maintenance, and mowing the lawn, there were suddenly relatives coming over to see the baby, doctor's appointments, meals to make, bottles to fill, and schedules to maintain. Amid the hectic rush of parenthood, some things just fell off the priority list. "Me time" was one of them. I'm sure you've been there, so you can understand that when it came to choosing between an extra hour of undisturbed sleep or going to the gym at 6:00 AM, I'm not ashamed to say I chose the comfort of my bed.

Skipping the gym was only the beginning. While I certainly knew better, I started eating whenever my son ate, and those of you who have kids know babies always have something in their mouths. So, as I'd give my son a cracker, some Cheerios, or a cookie, I'd help myself to a handful. Of course, grazing on my son's snacks wasn't the only dietary change. Because our schedules were so tight, my wife and I often ordered pizza or brought home takeout instead of making the healthy meals we did pre-baby.

The Shocking Moment of Truth

Then, on my son's second birthday, it hit me. After my son had gone to bed, I polished off the leftover French fries from his plate, sliced myself a second serving of birthday cake, and joined my in-laws to watch the video of our son's "first day" in the hospital.

About halfway through the video, my mother-in-law exclaimed, "Wow, Mike, it looks like you put on more than a few sympathy pounds since the birth. Never thought you'd end up a chubby hubby."

Everyone laughed and I let the comment slide, but deep down I was shocked. I knew I had gained a few pounds, but I didn't think it was *that* noticeable. Besides, I didn't feel fat. Sure, most of my clothes no longer fit, but I was pretty sure my muscle tone was still there underneath the rolls. All I needed was a week at the gym. Yup, after a couple of intense workouts, I would drop those few extra pounds I had gained and be back to my buff self.

But then I made the fatal mistake. I asked my wife if she noticed my weight gain. She responded with, "There's just more of you to love," combined with a sympathy pat on my rounded tummy.

That was it. The moment of truth had arrived. As soon as everyone left, I pulled out the bathroom scale. *More of me to love . . . What was my wife talking about?* I looked down and there it was: the fateful number. But I hadn't gained just a few pounds like I thought. I had gained a whopping 50 pounds in two years!

Standing on the scale and looking into the mirror, I realized I had become what I promised I would never be: fat. My mother-in-law was right. I was a chubby hubby. I had to do something about it—*fast*—or 50 pounds might become 60 or 70.

While it was clear that I was on the road to Fat Town, I was still a dad, without any extra time to work out or the money to hire a personal chef to prepare healthy meals. I also wasn't about to spend time counting calories, measuring out servings, or calculating my daily carb and fat intake. I needed something simple that fit into my already-packed day; most of all, I needed something that worked.

Dad fat: *n.* the extra weight and responsibility of fatherhood converted into body mass. Also known as blubber; dreaded spare-tire gut. *See also* chubby hubby.

Losing the Dad Fat

Time is one of the most valuable things parents have, and once you add one or two kids into the equation, you soon realize there is never enough of it. But becoming a dad does more than take away time. One study released by Duke University Medical Center found that in addition to a change in eating habits and exercise, other physiological factors also occurred once children appeared on the scene. While the study can't explain exactly why the 4,523 fathers involved in the research gained the weight, they did find the risk of obesity went up by 4 percent and that number grew as the couple had more children.

Standing on the scale and barely able to read the number over my bulging stomach, I had to admit I had become one of these men. But there was no way I was going to stay that way. I decided at that moment that I would take my expertise in nutrition and fitness and devise a way to increase my cardiovascular level, reduce my body fat, and get toned—all in less than an hour a day.

I wish I could say the answer came to me overnight, but it didn't happen that way. The core of the *Buff Dad* program came to me as I was watching my wife talk on the phone while emptying the dishwasher, carrying my son, and cleaning up the kitchen. The solution was to multitask. In order for a weight-loss program to accomplish everything I wanted, all of the components had to be synchronized to work at the same time.

But there was one other important factor I needed to take into consideration. I wanted the program to work—not just for a few weeks, but for the rest of my life. I didn't want to be a fat dad today, and I was pretty sure I didn't want to be one again two years, five years, or even ten years down the line. My plan had to have something that helped me not only lose weight, but also help boost my metabolism and keep me continuously burning calories in the long run.

Combining my nutritional background with research in exercise physiology, I created a plan that took advantage of every man's secret weapon when it comes to weight loss: our testosterone.

One of the great things about being a guy is that our testosterone is already built in as part of our chemical makeup. While it helps us in the bedroom, it also provides a big advantage when it comes to weight loss. Aside from making us our manly selves, testosterone helps build more muscle quickly, which increases our metabolism and our ability to burn more fat.

You've probably read or seen in the news stories about pro athletes who pump themselves up with testosterone injections in order to build muscle and look lean, but two other healthier ways to do the same thing are often overlooked.

The first way is to eat foods that naturally help build the amount of testosterone surging through your body without negative side effects. By eating more testosterone-rich foods, you'll crank up your resting metabolism naturally and burn more fat. The good news is that most of the foods are normal items you can find in the grocery store. You'll learn more about the top-ten testosterone powerfoods and how to add them to your diet using the *Buff Dad* Dietary Plan in Chapter 3.

The second way to boost your body's testosterone levels is by exercising, but before you pop in a cardio tape and start sweating to the oldies, there's one important thing you need to know: not all exercise will give you the results you want.

Through my research and years of training professional athletes, I've learned the most effective form of exercise is strength training. Keeping the goal of multitasking to get faster results, I developed a special supersetting workout to help you lose your fat-dad poundage quickly and keep it off without starving yourself or spending hours in the gym. I've found that when working out this way, you not only increase your metabolism as you build more muscle, but you tone up while you do it—killing two problems with one activity.

Using the *Buff Dad* workout, you'll get results twice as fast as doing only cardio or only weight lifting. This is because the program takes the idea of multitasking a step further by combining several strength-training exercises to "overwork" the muscles while providing an aerobic workout. In other words, you're working out faster and doing both aerobics and strength training at one time. I'll cover this more in Chapter 7 when I take you through the *Buff Dad* Workout Blitz.

Of course, when you're not working out, you'll be feeding your body testosterone-rich foods that, when combined with the workout, will help you produce more lean muscle mass, increase bone density, and improve other aspects of your life that your wife will also enjoy.

Using both the diet and the workout together, you'll get double the results without doubling the time it takes or the effort involved.

What You Can Expect from the *Buff Dad* Program

Once I started the *Buff Dad* program, I noticed results right away—and I wasn't the only one. My wife noticed the change in me, too. My body was changing, but so was my energy level and my attitude. I was more positive and had a better outlook on life. While losing weight was one of the reasons for my new upbeat personality, some scientists are now suggesting that healthy testosterone levels can also help improve a guy's mood.

Plus, because I was working out, I slept better at night and was able to think more clearly during the day. It was as if shedding 50 pounds of dad fat put me back in the fast lane of life—physically, personally, and mentally.

By following the four-week *Buff Dad* program, you will get the results you want, too. You'll see incredible changes in just twenty-eight days. Of course, depending on how much weight you need to lose, not everyone will reach their ideal goal in one month and will need to continue for a longer period of time. But unlike some fad or drastic calorie-reduction programs that are unhealthy to continue indefinitely, my program gives you the tools you need to keep going until you reach your own ideal body weight.

The *Buff Dad* program also works for men of all ages—whether you're a young father in his twenties or a dad in his late forties.

Regardless of your age, the program helps men build muscle, lose fat, and increase testosterone levels. After four weeks, you'll have more energy, more virility, and more tone. The only thing the program doesn't combat is male-pattern baldness. Sorry, but you're on your own with that one.

Most important, the program comes with a maintenance plan. After putting in the time and effort to become buff, the last thing you're going to want is to gain it all back. The *Buff Dad* program is not a get-fit-quick program but one that teaches you how to incorporate fitness and healthy eating into your hectic life so you can enjoy fatherhood even more. I strongly believe being "buff" is more than building muscle. It's a lifestyle that affects you physically, mentally, and emotionally.

Whether you're ready for it or not, your life is about to change for the better. Let's get started.

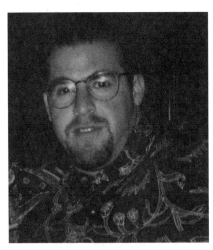

From a puffy daddy....

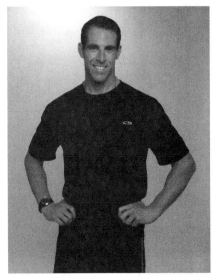

To a buff daddy. Me, sixty pounds lighter and leaner.

CHAPTER 2

THE TESTOSTERONE ADVANTAGE

Understanding the Power Behind the Program

The man who goes the furthest is generally the one who is willing to do and dare.

Dale Carnegie

A ccording to the International Health, Racquet and Sports Club Association (IHRSA), more than 33.8 million Americans worked out in a health club in 2001, and the number of health clubs and gyms in the United States increased consistently between the years of 1998 and 2002. The question is, if so many of us have been working out, why are we still fat?

For years, fitness experts and nutritionists have been telling us we had to eat less and work out more. They've also been telling us that to be classified as fit, you either had to look like you were ready to compete in a weight-lifting competition or do hours of cardio exercise. Guess what? They were wrong. A study reported in *Biological Psychiatry* in May 2007 showed that low-fat dieting can increase stress levels, and some research proves that hours of cardio may not be as effective as we once thought. In fact, hours of weekly endurance work may deflate and weaken fast-twitch muscles, making it harder to build strength.

So what should we be doing? We should be working out *less* and eating foods that work *for* our bodies. In other words, we need to work out smarter. By using testosterone to your advantage, you can achieve both of those things.

Testosterone: The Good, the Bad, and the Science of Becoming Buff

As men, we have one advantage over women when it comes to losing weight: our testosterone. Studies from the *American Journal of Physiology* prove that an increase in testosterone levels has a direct correlation on lean muscle mass. In other words, more testosterone means more muscle mass, which leads to a higher metabolism and less body fat. As a result, we can lose weight faster and keep it off longer than women can. (My wife thinks this is completely unfair, but if there's any advantage to losing weight quickly and effectively, I'm all for it.)

I know what you're probably thinking: *If testosterone is already pumping through my body naturally, then how did I get fat?* The answer might surprise you.

Are You Man Enough? The Steady Decline of the Big T

The first big shocker is that Father Time has it in for us. You would think that being one of the "big dads" of the universe, he would be sympathetic and even help us out, but that's not the case.

You see, even though I'm not quite forty and I'm healthy overall, the testosterone in my body is already decreasing, and has been doing so for years. I'm in a downward spiral, and things are only going to get worse.

Now before you start to feel sorry for me, I have news for you: this downward spiral happens to every man. Sadly, our body's production of the manly hormone starts to decline earlier than we may have thought. Research conducted at ZRT Laboratory in Beaverton, Oregon, found that men peak in testosterone production in their early twenties and sharply decline after that. Most men can expect their testosterone to drop by about 1 percent a year beginning in their fifties, which means that by the time you're seventy, you'll have only half the testosterone you had at twenty-five.

While this sounds bad enough, there is even more bad news. A Massachusetts Male Aging Study, reported in the *Journal of Clinical Endocrinology and Metabolism,* revealed that men are losing their testosterone faster than those in older generations. Studying 1,709 men born between 1916 and 1945, researchers noticed the younger men in the study had surprisingly low testosterone levels. In fact, a sixty-year-old in 2003 had about 15 percent less testosterone than a man who was sixty in 1988. In other words, sixty was looking like the new seventy. So what does that do for us men who are only in our thirties? At forty, will our bodies be producing the same testosterone as our sixty-year-old grandfathers?

The Big T Decline: Why It's Happening

Research isn't sure exactly when our bodies stop producing testosterone altogether, but they do know it slowly depletes, causing a reduction in lean muscle mass, a loss of energy, and a decrease in our sex drive. A study reported in *Environmental Health Perspectives* showed that, in general, testosterone levels seem to be on a steady decline worldwide, dropping by a whopping 1 percent a year.

The really bad news for American dads is that declining testosterone is the worst in the United States, which is probably why those little blue pills are so wildly popular and you see all those erectile dysfunction (ED) commercials on TV.

Big T Decline	
United States: –68%*	Denmark: –20%
Brazil: –45%	Nigeria: –10%
Israel: –34%	Finland: +8%
Hong Kong: –30%	Sweden: +15%
France: –26%	Germany: +16%

Based on sperm concentrations between 1934 and 1996. Source: "Testosterone Under Attack," Men's Health, September 2007.

Now before you pack your bags and move to Sweden or one of the other few countries where the Big T is on the rise, one explanation for the drastic testosterone decline in the majority of countries could be that we are now fatter. According to Thomas G. Travison, Ph.D., the lead author of the Massachusetts Male Aging Study, obesity is a powerful indicator of low testosterone. If your body mass index (BMI) goes up by 10 percent, your testosterone drops by the same percentage. As a result, fat dads like us have approximately 25 percent less testosterone surging through our bodies than fit guys, and without testosterone, we lose muscle tone, which means we burn less calories and we end up getting fatter . . . thus losing even more testosterone. It's like a never-ending circle of doom.

The *Buff Dad* program puts this cycle into reverse. First, it gets rid of fat, which makes you look good. Second, it helps boost testosterone within your body so you feel good, have more energy, and can keep your spouse happy, too.

But don't worry. Just because you're increasing your testosterone, you will not look like those massive weight-lifting guys in the gym. You know who they are: the guys so bulked up they can't see their toes over their massive chests and have to wear MC Hammer pants because their thighs are so large they no longer can squeeze into normal jeans. The *Buff Dad* program is designed to firm your body, help you lose inches of flab, and increase your lean muscle mass—not turn you into the Incredible Hulk.

Testosterone Myths: Tackling the Scare Factor

We've all heard the horror stories. Testosterone will turn you into a mean killing machine and then you'll die. Thankfully this only happens in high dosages, and the chances of it occurring are pretty rare. Besides, solid scientific proof that the Big T causes violent outbursts has not been proven. If it were true, all men, because we naturally have testosterone in our bodies, would be on the verge of going crazy. Of course, if you ask my wife, there are days she's convinced I'm already there—like the time I ordered the X-treme fire chicken wings and then ate the whole basket just to prove to her I could—even though they were so spicy, I thought my lips were going to burn off.

So before you start thinking you're about to become a ticking time bomb, keep in mind that many of the superbuff men you see in Wrestling Mania and other sports injected themselves with the hormone. Building testosterone naturally through food and exercise is completely different from pumping it into your body through a needle. By eating more proteins and healthy fats, your body will convert those foods into *usable* testosterone. In other words, you're not force-feeding the muscles, as the body only utilizes what it needs.

Think of the *Buff Dad* program as a way to enhance your body's natural functions. You might have already figured this out with your own nonscientific study, but as men, we generate testosterone in a twenty-four-hour cycle. While none of us have exactly the same cycle, there is a certain time of day that we peak. For many of us, this is in the early morning. Then we continue through the day, using up our testosterone, and peak again the next day. Just like a marathon runner who needs to replenish his carbs on a daily basis, we need to make sure our testosterone is in steady supply so that we continuously keep our lean muscle mass and burn more calories.

The Health Benefits
of Natural Testosterone

By enhancing your testosterone levels, you'll also be improving your health, and I don't just mean your sexual health. Numerous studies, including one reported in *Arteriosclerosis and Thrombosis,* showed that by raising testosterone levels, men were actually able to decrease their "bad" LDL cholesterol and improve their "good" HDL cholesterol. Another study performed at London's National Heart & Lung Institute showed that increasing testosterone levels in men over fifty helped improve blood flow and oxygen to the heart, even in men who had a history of heart disease.

Testosterone plays a role in how we utilize our oxygen, balance our blood sugar, regulate cholesterol, and maintain our overall neurological functions. In other words, it helps keep you healthy, thinking clearly, and feeling happy. Most importantly, in terms of helping you with your weight-loss goals, it builds muscle.

But that's not all. The other bonus about increasing your testosterone naturally is the absence of scary side effects. You won't have to worry about unusual hair loss or acne outbreaks, and you definitely won't have any of the embarrassing side effects that you get from taking ED pills, such as erections that last for six hours. While research shows steroid use is associated with heart disease, cancer, liver damage, and other life-shortening conditions, there are no negative side effects from increasing your testosterone stores naturally.

However, there is one other side effect you'll encounter and one that your wife may notice—although I doubt she's going to complain. With more testosterone coursing through your body, you may find you'll have improved sexual function, which works out as an extra bonus for dads like me who are in their thirties and are already past their sexual prime.

Buff Dad Secret #1:
How to Maximize Testosterone with Fuel

When I first started trying to lose my 50 pounds of dad fat, I admit I attempted taking what I thought was the easy way out: cutting back on my calories, reducing my fat intake, and eliminating as many carbohydrates as possible. I basically ate nothing but salad.

Within a week, I had lost a measly 5 pounds, along with my energy and my sense of humor. While losing 5 pounds isn't bad and falls within the generally accepted healthy rate of losing weight (2 to 5 pounds is average), after the torture I had gone through, I had expected to lose more. Keep in mind, I wanted to lose 50 pounds, so living on salad and feeling like crap for the next ten weeks wasn't something I was looking forward to going through. Besides, I was tired all the time, I couldn't think straight, and the smallest of obstacles would frustrate me. Something as simple as "Honey, could you fix the dripping faucet in the upstairs bathroom?" would send my brain into a panic mode. I couldn't focus.

Needless to say, my wife wasn't impressed with the new "slightly lighter and still squishy" me and couldn't wait for me to fall off the diet wagon. And I did fall, ten days later, gaining back 5 pounds in two days. Why did I fail on my first dieting attempt? Because I cut out all the testosterone foods my body needed.

Going low-fat is the *worst* thing you can do as a guy. Research reported in the *Journal of Applied Physiology* revealed that low-fat diets don't work for men because they suppress the manufacture of testosterone—the main weapon we have to help us lose weight. Your body *needs* fat to manufacture testosterone. Without it, your testosterone levels go down, and you reduce your ability to burn muscle, burn fat, and keep your wife happy—in more ways than just being less grouchy.

But there is good news. The best fats for building testosterone are the same unsaturated and omega-3 fats that make you feel full longer. You won't be hungry on the *Buff Dad* program, and because you're not hungry, you won't feel like you're on a diet. You also won't feel the need to "cheat" or go back to your old ways. Instead, you'll be able to continuously stay on the *Buff Dad* program and incorporate it into your daily life.

In addition to good fats, there are other Big T powerfoods that supercharge your testosterone levels. While some of them include vegetables, such as broccoli and cabbage, other mouth-watering foods like steak, burgers, pasta, and chili also play a key role in helping you get buff by increasing your testosterone. One final piece of good news is that many of the foods you need to boost your testosterone are foods you probably have in your refrigerator already, and if you don't have them, they are easily accessible.

However, it's going to take a little bit more than chowing down with testosterone-enhancing foods to transform you from your chubby-hubby state to a buff dad your spouse won't be able to resist. That's where the *Buff Dad* Workout Blitz comes in.

Buff Dad Secret #2:
Releasing Testosterone Through Exercise

When my wife was pregnant, I used to have these "dad and son" fantasies about how my life was going to be. One of them was the "jogging dream." The plan was that I would get up early every morning, place my son in one of those jogger strollers, and go for an hour-long run. In my mind, it was like a Hollywood movie. Pushing my son, I would jog down the street, waving at my neighbors going to work and the paperboy delivering the morning news. Of course, I wouldn't be huffing and puffing, but looking like an Olympian.

Needless to say, this never happened. And after I'd put on the 50 pounds of dad fat, I wouldn't have been able to go very far without being winded.

The good news is that aerobics wouldn't have helped me become buff. Sure, it's great exercise if you want to strengthen your heart and lungs, and it will help you burn fat, but really it does nothing for the rest of your body. In other words, it won't make you buff.

Research shows that to lose one pound you have to burn 3,500 calories, but the average person only burns 100 calories per mile. I don't know about you, but I wanted a faster way to burn calories that could easily fit into my schedule and make me look good at the same time—remember, the *Buff Dad* program is all about multitasking.

Besides, even if I did have the time to run for hours, I'd eventually end up burning away both my muscle tone and my fat. I'd be thinner, but not toned. Plus, depending on my genetic and physical makeup, I could damage my joints and put unnecessary stress on my body.

I'm not saying endurance exercises are bad. I'm just saying there are better ways to get the body and tone you want without having to run for hours every day. The most effective way to build muscle is through weight training and doing a little bit of cardio. For every pound of fat you have, you burn 6 calories a day. Muscle, on the other hand, burns an incredible 50 calories a day—that's eight times more calories. That's why on the *Buff Dad* program you'll be doing a little of both: some weight lifting and some cardio, but only enough cardio to effectively burn fat. You'll learn more about this in Chapter 5.

BUFF FACT

Every pound of muscle you have burns approximately 50 calories a day. Every pound of fat burns only about 6 calories a day.

So what does testosterone have to do with weight training? Everything—at least when it comes to losing weight and looking good—and I'm not the only one who knows this.

In 1999, the School of Exercise Science and Sports Management at Southern Cross University in Lismore, Australia, conducted tests on twenty-one weight trainers to see how testosterone affected the body. Their research showed improvements in lean-tissue mass, arm girth, and thigh circumference. But what really surprised the researchers was how testosterone affected the men who had flabby stomachs. Based on their skin-fold measurements, these men lost a significant number of inches from their waists. Basically, these guys were able to say good-bye to their love handles and hello to firm abs.

This is only the beginning. Researchers at the Charles R. Drew University of Medicine and Science in Los Angeles combined testosterone supplementation in HIV-infected men who had declining levels of natural testosterone. The results were surprising. In the thirty-four-month study, all the men given testosterone added more than 5 pounds of muscle, even the men who did not lift a single weight during the entire time.

This news is great if you're the lazy type, because even if you're lax on going to the gym, at least eating to increase your testosterone is going to help you out. Of course, if you want to be buff, you'll need to do some weight lifting and a bit of cardio to burn off the fat.

What about age? What if you're over thirty years old, have been in the downhill spiral for a while, and haven't been producing a lot of testosterone naturally? According to some recent research, age doesn't matter.

In a study reported in *The Journal of Clinical Endocrinology and Metabolism*, researchers found that older men were just as responsive as younger men to testosterone doses in building muscle-mass. The study took sixty healthy older men (ages sixty to seventy-five) and sixty-one younger men (ages eighteen to thirty-four) and compared the relationship of testosterone and muscle mass building in each of the groups. After twenty weeks of regulating their testosterone, the researchers tested the men's muscles based on exercises that included leg press strength, leg press power, and leg press fatigability.

They also tested the guys' physical performance based on stair-climbing, a ten-meter walk, and timed up-and-go. All assessments were conducted at the beginning and end of the study, and results were evaluated based on age and testosterone dosage.

What they learned was that it didn't matter whether the subject was eighteen years old or seventy years old: all men demonstrated significant changes in muscle strength. In fact, the older men had the same muscular changes as the younger men.

While the tests proved how testosterone increased muscle, they also showed that testosterone had no effect on the men's physical functions, such as their ability to climb more stairs or walk faster. In other words, if you want to run a marathon, don't count on testosterone to get you there, but if you want to be buff, testosterone is the way to go.

More tests on testosterone were done at the University of Rome, confirming that men with high testosterone could work out longer. During the testing process, researchers discovered the muscle fibers of men who had more testosterone tended not to fatigue as quickly as normal- or low-testosterone men. In other words, if you had more testosterone in your body, you could work out harder and longer—giving you a much bigger advantage over other men. Plus, because you are working out harder, you'll need to work out less to get the same results.

So, if this concept appeals to you, it's time to get started on the way to newfound buffness. In Chapter 4, you'll learn what foods you should eat. Chapter 7 will take you through the *Buff Dad* Workout Blitz. Plus, you can find more tips at www.buffdads.com.

PART II

GETTING STARTED

CHAPTER 3

UNDERSTANDING YOUR BODY AND THE FOOD YOU EAT

If you are what you eat, and you don't know what you are eating, then do you know who you are?

Claude Fischler

I f you're like me, you've probably been on a diet at some point in your life, so unfortunately you know what that entails. Usually it means you'll be feeling hungry for a few days or even a few weeks and then bingeing at the end on fast food and high-fat desserts.

You've probably also figured out that diets don't work. If they did, you wouldn't be reading this book. One thing to keep in mind is the *Buff Dad* Dietary Plan is not a diet. In fact, if you compare it to diets you've been on in the past, you could almost say it's the anti-diet. That's because you won't be hungry, and you will lose weight.

MythBuster #1:
The Problem with Popular Diets

W e've all heard the rules: Don't eat carbs. Don't eat fat. Don't eat sugar. Don't eat red meat. Really, if you cut out all those foods, what's left?

Imagine living without pizza, cheese, hamburgers, ice cream, or any of your other favorite foods for the rest of your life. I don't know about you, but I really love to eat, and not just carrot sticks and salads. I don't care what anyone says, but a diet is doomed to fail if you're never allowed to eat the things that you love. Don't even get me started on these 1,200-calories-a-day meal plans. Not only do they affect you physically, but they affect you mentally. One recent diet I looked into said you could expect anything from abdominal cramping to irritability while following their meal plan. I couldn't believe it. I have to be hungry, in pain, and grouchy just to lose a few lousy pounds? I don't think so.

The main problem with many trendy diets is that they work only for a short time. Sure, you might lose 10 pounds in a week on the maple syrup, cabbage soup, or grapefruit diet, but as soon as you go back to eating normally, you'll end up gaining it all back—and then some.

The reason we gain the weight back is that our body really hates being hungry. When we diet, our body thinks the world suddenly ran out of food and kicks into antistarvation mode.

Of course, we know we won't starve, especially if we're already overweight, but our bodies don't take fat percentage into account. It doesn't matter whether you are 10 pounds below your ideal weight, 10 pounds overweight, or morbidly obese, the body responds in the same manner. The body gets hungry. It decides it needs to conserve energy, which it accomplishes by slowing down your metabolism. Strange as it sounds, you need to eat to lose weight healthily.

Moreover, when you're eating less, not only are you burning fewer calories, but half the calories you do burn come from lean muscle tissue. Let me tell you a secret: you don't want to lose muscle. First of all, you want to be a buff dad and not a scrawny dad; second, muscle burns more calories than fat. In other words, the more muscle you have, the more calories you burn even when you're doing nothing at all.

Remember that each pound of muscle you have burns about 50 calories a day, so if you add a pound of muscle, you burn more calories. Unfortunately, it also works the other way. If you starve your body and lose a pound of muscle, your metabolism slows down by 50 calories a day and you're stuck in a catch-up phase. You'll have to eat less to compensate for the slower metabolism; you'll then lose more muscle and have to eat even fewer calories in order to lose weight. The bottom line: skip the starvation diets.

MythBuster #2: The Food Pyramid

Back in grade school, we were taught about the Food Pyramid. You know the one: a big base of carbohydrates on the bottom, fruits and veggies in the middle, then the smaller servings of protein, and finally the tiny bit of fat at the top. The good news is this old-fashioned pyramid has been revised twice—once in 1992 and again in 2005. But there is one big problem with the pyramid. It's wrong for our processed and pre-prepared eating lifestyle.

While the pyramid is a great starting point to make the general public aware of what they should eat, it really only works if foods are simple, such as fruit, meat, grains, and fat. What if you are eating a mix of these categories? How do you classify them? There are more processed foods, high-fat foods, and sugary foods available than ever before. Even when trying to be healthy today, there's a good chance you're still eating some sort of processed addition. Look at microwave popcorn. You think you're being "good" by buying a low-fat snack only to discover it's covered in trans fat and then coated with sugar. (Why do you think Kettle Corn is so sweet?) This food not only counts as a carbohydrate on the Food Pyramid, but it would also increase your daily fat and sugar consumption.

Saying Good-Bye to Fat Dad Forever

For optimal results on the *Buff Dad* program, the average 200- to 250-pound guy should eat 2,000 calories a day. I could give you absolute calculations of how much protein, carbs, and fat you should be eating, but you don't have time to worry about the numbers behind what you're putting into your mouth all day long. Instead, I've designed the *Buff Dad* Dietary Plan (see Chapter 6 for full details) to make sure you are getting roughly the right percentage of each component and the right number of calories. All you have to do is follow the plan.

Your *Buff Dad* Daily Calorie Intake

150–200 pounds—1,800 calories

200–250 pounds—2,000 calories

250–300 pounds—2,200 calories

300–350 pounds—2,400 calories

350+ pounds—2,600 calories

What makes the *Buff Dad* Dietary Plan different from other plans is that not only can you stay on the program for the rest of your life, but the plan is focused on improving your testosterone levels. You already know testosterone is what makes you different from your wife and makes you the man you are today, but what you may not know is how it affects your physique and why it's important if you want to be buff.

Unlike those myths that claim testosterone will turn you into the Hulk, the hormone doesn't actually work that way unless you happen to be injecting massive doses of it into your butt. What it does do when ingested properly is convert more of your muscle fibers from the type that give you energy to those that grow big. In other words, you're transforming your skinny arms into ones that look toned. Without testosterone's help in switching up the fibers, your muscle girth would be limited. Just think about women: no matter how much they lift, they never get as big as a guy. They don't have the magic of testosterone coursing through their bodies.

Testosterone also prevents muscle degradation. When your body gets hungry and needs more energy, it pulls protein from your muscles and shrinks them, an unfortunate effect, especially when you've been working so hard. You want to look good, and you want your hours in the gym to pay off. You don't want your muscles to disappear whenever your body needs an extra shot of protein.

The good news is that testosterone stops this from happening. Instead, your body will pull protein from other areas of the body before going to the muscles. Of course, if you follow the *Buff Dad* Dietary Plan, you'll be getting more than enough testosterone, so you'll never have to worry about this problem.

BUFF FACT

According to the *American Journal of Clinical Nutrition,* people who ate six times a day had a faster resting heartbeat than those who ate three times a day.

Eat More to Lose Weight

When should you eat? The answer is six times a day or every three hours. While you might have been brought up believing in three big meals a day, eating more frequently is actually better for you. Not only are you never hungry, but because your body is always digesting, it never goes into starvation mode. Your metabolism is constantly working to digest food and burn body fat.

In fact, a report published in the *European Journal of Clinical Nutrition* found that people who ate six times a day had a faster resting metabolic rate than those who ate three times a day. Another study found that those poor people who only ate three times a day also ended up with more body fat when compared to those who ate more often.

Here's the short version: the more often you eat, presuming you're eating the right foods, the more calories you burn.

CHAPTER 4

WHAT TO EAT ON THE *BUFF DAD* PROGRAM

One's destination is never a place but rather a new way of looking at things.

Henry Miller

It's now time to cut through all the confusion and get your diet back on track.

In this chapter, I outline all the foods you need to eat in order to get buff. All you have to do is follow along and be committed. Yes, *committed*. I'm not saying you'll never get to eat fattening foods again, but for the next four weeks, you need to be committed to making some changes about how and what you eat.

Thankfully, you won't have to change everything, but you may need to change some core components because, let's face it, what you've been doing up until this point hasn't been working. But don't worry— the *Buff Dad* Dietary Plan isn't rocket science. At the end of the book, I've included more than thirty easy-to-prepare recipes along with a four-week meal plan to get you started. You'll also find more helpful tips on the Buff Dad website, www.buffdads.com. The recipes are simple and easy to make, and in most cases they require less than thirty minutes to prepare. Plus, because meals are not restricted to any food groups, you can still have a normal family mealtime.

The Top-Ten Testosterone Powerfoods

To make it easy for you, the *Buff Dad* Dietary Plan already includes the ten testosterone powerfoods. This way you won't have to worry about getting your daily dose. Plus, if you don't like the plan and want to make your own meals, the recipes I've included at the end of the book also use a wide range of these powerfoods.

But if you happen to create your own snacks or order out while on the program, you should keep a few powerfoods in mind when making your selections. Ten foods that boost testosterone levels naturally and help develop more muscle tone are as follows.

1 Lean Beef

What's Inside: Protein, iron, magnesium, zinc, saturated fat.

The Facts: "Few things have as positive an impact on testosterone levels as lean meats," says Larrian Gillespie, retired assistant urology professor and author of many health and nutrition books. Beef specifically offers the added benefit of having high protein and zinc—two nutrients key to optimizing testosterone and muscle-building potential—in one source. While too much saturated fat is not a good thing, you require some to produce testosterone.

How to Get It: Grill or broil a lean cut of steak a few times a week.

2 Beans
....

What's Inside: Protein, fiber, zinc.

The Facts: Beans pack a bigger shot of zinc than any other member of the veggie family; some (like baked beans) even rival the zinc content of red meat. Add it to a food that's high in protein and fiber and low in fat, and you have a winning combo.

How to Get It: Baked beans, lima beans, navy beans, and kidney beans are all good choices. Canned versions are just as nutritious as dry.

3 Poultry
....

What's Inside: Protein and little fat.

The Facts: "High-protein diets have a positive impact on muscle mass and thus testosterone levels," says John E. Morley, director of the Division of Geriatric Medicine at St. Louis University. "High fat has the opposite effect." So while chicken and turkey lack high zinc levels, their protein-to-fat ratios make them important to your diet.

How to Get It: Roast or grill skinless, boneless portions of turkey or chicken several times a week. Or choose chicken and turkey cold cuts for lunch.

4 Eggs *(preferably egg whites)*

What's Inside: Protein and cholesterol.

The Facts: "Testosterone is synthesized from cholesterol, and as such, food containing cholesterol is a good source of building blocks for testosterone," says Robert S. Tan, M.D., associate professor of geriatric medicine and andrologist at the University of Texas in Houston. (An andrologist specializes in male diseases, especially those affecting the male reproductive system.) Eggs are a source of pure, unadulterated cholesterol, and one recent study shows that the excess cholesterol in eggs isn't as harmful as previously thought.

How to Get It: Start your day with three or four eggs or egg whites cooked in olive oil or fat-free cooking spray. Egg whites are lower in calories and are recommended in most of the *Buff Dad* recipes.

5 Cottage Cheese *(1 percent milk fat)*

What's Inside: Protein with very little fat.

The Facts: One cup of 1 percent cottage cheese has more protein and less fat than a serving of lean beef or chicken. Have it as a snack or with a meal for testosterone-boosting potential.

How to Get It: Eat 1 cup of cottage cheese each day. Add 1 teaspoon of cinnamon for extra flavor.

6 Broccoli

What's Inside: Indole-3-carbinol, fiber.

The Facts: "Elevated estrogen levels lead to fat accumulation and can interfere with muscle growth," says Chris Aceto, author of *Championship Bodybuilding*. In a clinical study, indole-3-carbinol found in broccoli reduced the female hormone estradiol by 50 percent in men, resulting in increased lean muscle and decreased fat.

How to Get It: Eat as many servings of broccoli as you can stomach.

7 Cabbage

What's Inside: Indole-3-carbinol, fiber.

The Facts: In addition to exhibiting the same estradiol-restricting properties as other cruciferous vegetables, cabbage is high in fiber. Because fiber is satisfying, you eat less overall. Moreover, keeping weight down has an anti-estrogen impact.

How to Get It: Load up that fat-free brat with sauerkraut and have a side of slaw. (Just go easy on the mayo.)

8 Brussels Sprouts

What's Inside: Indole-3-carbinol, fiber.

The Facts: Listen to your mom: Brussels sprouts do help you grow up big and strong. Like the other vegetables on the list, Brussels sprouts specifically target bad estrogen and pack in the fiber.

How to Get It: Hold your nose and power them down.

9 Garlic

What's Inside: Allicin (an enzyme produced within the clove).

The Facts: In clinical studies, garlic's active ingredient, allicin, enhances testosterone levels and inhibits cortisol, a hormone that competes with testosterone by limiting its actions and breaking down muscle tissue.

How to Get It: Season other foods with garlic, but eating whole cloves provides the most direct benefit.

10 Oysters

What's Inside: Protein, magnesium, lots of zinc.

The Facts: Along with increasing physical endurance, oysters pack more zinc than almost any other food source. Just six oysters give you almost seven times the recommended daily allowance of zinc, and zinc plays a key role in muscle growth and testosterone levels.

How to Get It: Eat a serving of oysters once a week—raw, cooked, or canned (preferably not fried).

BUFF FACT

Cinnamon helps curb sugar cravings and hunger by increasing the transit of glucose to the brain.

Building Your Meals the
Buff Dad Way

So, should you eat only the top-ten powerfoods? Of course not. You need a mix of proteins, carbs, and vegetables. While the powerfoods are the ones that help boost your testosterone, you need more than the Big T to be healthy. You still need calcium, vitamins, and other nutrients to make your entire body run like a well-oiled machine.

Losing weight and becoming buff aren't complicated. In fact, it's as simple as 1–2–3 because each of your meals on the *Buff Dad* Dietary Plan consists of one food from each of the three columns:

One	One	One
lean protein	carbohydrate	high-fiber vegetable

NOTE: *If you really hate veggies, you only need to add them to two of your meals.*

The secret behind the *Buff Dad* foods is not only what you eat, but how much of everything you eat. I'm not talking about measuring and weighing all your food. Instead of wasting your time with cups and scales, to get the maximum testosterone benefits, it's better to eat in thirds: a third of carbs, a third of high-fiber vegetables, and a third of lean protein.

Lean Proteins	Carbohydrates	Vegetables
Chicken or turkey breast	Baked potato	Broccoli
	Sweet potato	Asparagus
Lean ham	Yam	Lettuce
Lean ground turkey	Squash	Carrots
Swordfish	Pumpkin	Cauliflower
Orange roughy	Brown rice (steamed or boiled)	Green beans
Haddock and all other white fish, such as tilapia, sea bass, and mahimahi	Wild rice (steamed or boiled)	Green peppers, red peppers
		Mushrooms
Salmon	High-fiber pasta (at least 4–6 grams of fiber per serving)	Spinach
Tuna		Tomato
Crab and lobster	Oatmeal (not instant) and other grain cereals	Peas
Oysters		Brussels sprouts
Shrimp	Barley or quinoa	Artichoke
Top round steak	Beans	Cabbage
Top sirloin steak	Corn	Celery
Buffalo/ostrich and other lean wild game meats	Strawberries	Zucchini
	Melon, cantaloupe	Cucumber
	Apple	Onion
Low-fat peanut butter (all natural)	Orange, grapefruit, and other fruits	All green leafy vegetables, including kale, escarole, and Swiss chard
Eggs, egg whites, or substitutes	Fat-free yogurt	
Low-fat cottage cheese	Whole-wheat bread	
Tofu and low-fat cheese	All berries, including blueberries, blackberries, and cherries	

BUFF FACT

The average American only consumes 15 grams of fiber a day. Nutritionists recommend between 20 and 35 grams of fiber a day.

After reading the list of foods you're allowed to eat, I'm sure you're thinking *Okay, these don't look that scary.* In fact, I bet you're eating many of the items already. There are a couple of rules, though. No deep-frying anything on the chart, for example, nor are you allowed to smother everything in gravy, but you don't have to steam everything either.

In the next section of the book, I'll give you tips on what you can do to spice up your new meals. Plus, if you're looking for a total no-brainer solution, you can also follow the sample meal plans and recipes at the end of the book, or visit www.buffdads.com.

CHAPTER 5

PUTTING YOUR MEALS TOGETHER

Imagine that you are a masterpiece unfolding, every second of every day, a work of art taking form with every breath.

Thomas Crum

O ut of the three food categories on the *Buff Dad* Dietary Plan—lean protein, high-fiber carbs, and veggies—protein is the one that will help curb your appetite.

Protein is great because it makes you feel full quickly, which means you'll be less likely to overeat. Protein also helps speed up your metabolism, which is always a good thing when you want to lose weight. Plus, eating protein comes with an extra bonus. Because it takes more energy for the body to process, you're burning more calories just by eating it in comparison to carbohydrates or fats.

Scientists tell us that protein uses up to two and a half times more energy to digest than carbohydrates. Every time you eat a juicy steak, you're burning calories with every bite. Yes, this is really true, although the calories you burn aren't going to match what you burn during your *Buff Dad* workout.

In addition to burning tons of extra calories, protein helps deplete your glycogen stores.

Protein is also essential in building muscle. The right amount of protein combined with the right amount of exercise can increase your muscle tone dramatically by building new muscle and, more importantly, by repairing the muscles you already have.

Each time you lift weights, you cause microscopic tears in the muscle tissue. This sounds painful, but you won't even feel it. It's actually a good thing. The body uses the protein you eat to repair the torn cells, making the muscle stronger. That way the next time you go to the gym, you'll be able to lift a little bit more.

The body also uses protein after it runs out of glycogen, which usually happens when you're doing a really intense workout and is more likely to happen during cardio sessions. If you don't have enough stored protein for energy, the body will start pulling the protein used in your muscles, which is why many marathon runners are generally lean and not buff. They use up their stored protein and then are forced to use the protein stored in the muscle cells. To prevent this from happening, it's a good idea to make sure you eat enough protein every day.

The Best Protein to Eat

Here are your best choices when it comes to protein.

Poultry *(chicken and turkey)*

One of the staples of the *Buff Dad* Dietary Plan is poultry: chicken and turkey. Both are low in fat and full of protein, and they can be used in a lot of recipes. Ground chicken and turkey are also part of the plan; you can use them to make tacos, chili, meat loaf, and burgers.

Eat often: Roasted, broiled, baked, sautéed, marinated, and grilled poultry.

Avoid: Deep-fried poultry, creamy stews, or potpies; don't eat the skin and don't add gravy.

Fish and Shellfish

Fish and shellfish are great testosterone-enhancing foods, and you know that's always a good thing. Filled with healthy omega oils, they help curb your appetite and build muscle. Fish can be pan-seared, grilled, baked, or poached. To enhance the flavor, you can add spices such as a low-fat marinade, blackening spice, or lemon and dill. If you're really innovative in the kitchen, you can add the seafood to a spicy broth for Creole- or Thai-flavored soups. You could also try cooking your fish on a cedar plank. Salmon is especially tasty this way.

Be creative when cooking your fish. Fish tacos are a good alternative to ground beef, and so are sushi and seafood paella without the rice. If you do use rice, use brown or wild and remember to keep your serving to the size of a medium potato or your fist.

Eat often: Salmon, tuna, cod, haddock, halibut, perch, sea bass, snapper, crab, oysters, and lobster.

Avoid: Tartar sauce, battered fish, fried fish, baked stuffed fish, or seafood covered in a creamy or butter sauce.

Red Meat

One of the great things about the *Buff Dad* Dietary Plan is you actually get to eat red meat—lots of it. But there is one requirement: it has to be lean. We're talking top round cuts, top sirloin, shank, round, flank, and chuck. It you see any fat, cut it off.

Eat often: Roasted, grilled, or barbecued.

Avoid: Cuts of meat with obvious fat, fried meats, and steaks and other prepared meats covered with gravy or creamy sauces such as a béarnaise.

Low-Fat Cottage Cheese

Cottage cheese has become the staple of every low-fat diet on the market, and with good reason. Not only is it full of protein, but it also has amino acids, such as glutamine, which help support muscle metabolism. If you want to be a buff dad, you may consider spooning down a little here and there.

Eat often: Mix cottage cheese with fresh fruit, low-fat yogurt, or add it to diced cabbage and carrots to make a high-protein coleslaw.

Avoid: Cottage cheese filled with sugary processed fruits.

Eggs, Egg Whites, and Egg Substitutes

While being a buff dad doesn't require making Arnold Schwarzenegger blender drinks filled with wheat germ and raw eggs, I do recommend eggs or egg whites as a source of protein. Egg whites have fewer calories, so while you are losing weight, it's better to eat them rather than whole eggs. I recommend the product Eggology (see page 242). Once you have become buff and are following the plan to maintain the weight, you can have whole eggs.

Eat often: Omelets, scrambled eggs, boiled eggs, and poached eggs.

Avoid: Hollandaise sauce and cheese, eggs cooked in bacon fat, egg salad, and drive-through egg sandwiches such as those at McDonald's.

Getting Your Daily Carb Fix

Carbohydrates have received a bad rap over the years, but it wasn't the carbs that made me gain 50 pounds of fat. Instead, it was the types of carbohydrates I was eating. We often forget that carbohydrates don't just mean bread, snack foods, and cookies; they also include fruits, dairy products, and healthy foods such as oatmeal.

When I think back to what I was eating before I became a buff dad, I must admit I did eat an abundance of carbohydrates, but it wasn't my fault. Those pesky foods tricked me. You see, carbs—even the good ones like apples—raise your blood sugar and give you an instant high.

Instead of taking a lot of time to process through your body, like protein and fats do, carbohydrates start working right away. The problem is they also burn off right away, and then you want more. In other words, you're always in an up-and-down cycle where you're either flying happy or craving more of the sugary good stuff.

So if carbs are so addictive, why are they on the *Buff Dad* Dietary Plan? The easy answer is that our body needs them. First of all, keep in mind that not all carbohydrates are the same. You've got your doughnuts, and then you've got your fruit. Naturally, a doughnut is going to send your blood sugar off the scale and then send you plummeting into a deeper crash than would a bowl of cherries. So try to stay away from man-made carbs. Most of them contain a lot of sugar you don't need.

Second, in order to keep the rush under control, choose carbohydrates containing a lot of fiber, at least 2 grams of fiber per serving. The more fiber they have, the longer they'll stay in your stomach and the longer it will be between cravings. High-fiber choices such as bran, whole-wheat bread, and barley are also pretty good at keeping your colon clean and can help prevent cancer.

So now that I've got you eating the good carbs, here's why you need them. Remember how I said your muscles burn glycogen for energy? Well, the glycogen comes from carbohydrates.

Your body is constantly interacting with the foods you eat—either burning them for energy or storing them for later use. You use the carbs for energy, the protein to build muscles, and the fat to help build testosterone. When you combine these categories in the right amounts and with the *Buff Dad* Workout Blitz, you'll end up using the carb and fat reserves and won't need to dip into your protein reserves that are stored in your muscles.

One other thing to keep in mind is that the best time to eat carbs is right after your workout. This way your body will start using up the glycogen right away and stop using the protein in your muscles. Eating carbs then also helps make sure you burn them right away, rather than have them go into storage.

The Best Carbohydrates to Eat

Here are the best carbohydrates for the *Buff Dad* program.

Potatoes, Sweet Potatoes, Yams

Unlike a lot of fad diets on the market, on the *Buff Dad* Dietary Plan you're allowed to have carbohydrates—and that includes potatoes. Now, don't get too excited. You still have to control your portions and not chow down on a gigantic mountain of garlic mashed potatoes. An average portion size is a potato about the size of your fist.

Because sweet potatoes taste sweeter (thus the name), you might think they have more calories. They don't. They have the same amount of calories as a regular potato and you can prepare them pretty much the same way—boiled, baked, and microwaved.

Eat often: Baked; mashed with low-fat milk; cut into wedges and broiled in the oven with a little garlic powder, oregano, or chili powder sprinkled on top.

Avoid: Butter, sour cream, mashed potatoes made with cream, scalloped potatoes, French fries, and potato chips.

Brown Rice

Brown rice tastes just like white rice except it's a lot more filling and packed with a lot more protein. The reason it's more satisfying than white rice is that it's not as processed, which is why it's still brown. Because it's not as processed, your body takes longer to burn it, giving you more energy.

Eat often: Seasoned with chives, mushrooms, and other vegetables; steamed or boiled in a mixture of water and low-fat chicken broth. Sushi made with brown rice is also a good choice and a great way to incorporate your seafood intake.

Avoid: White rice, rice boiled with butter, fried rice.

Oatmeal

I feel like my mom when I say this, but eat your oatmeal! Oatmeal is a great carbohydrate. It's satisfying, quick to make (either at home or at work), and tastes good.

Eat often: With fresh fruit, NutraSweet, or cinnamon. Instead of using water, try adding low-fat yogurt to oatmeal. To make it more satisfying, add the oatmeal to the yogurt and let it sit overnight. The oats will swell as they absorb the moisture from the yogurt, and it will feel like you are eating more.

Avoid: Processed single-serving packages filled with sugar.

High-Fiber Pasta

If you are a pasta lover, don't despair. High-fiber pasta (at least 4–6 grams per serving) or whole-wheat pasta is perfect for the *Buff Dad* Dietary Plan. Just don't overdo it. There's a big difference between a serving of pasta (1 cup) and a heaping plate of creamy fettuccini Alfredo that could feed a family of four. Also, pasta shouldn't be eaten on its own. Always combine it with a protein.

Eat often: Plain, with tomato sauce, or with vegetables and lemon squeezed over it.

Avoid: Creamy Alfredo sauces, butter, white pasta, and most cheeses. You can sprinkle low-fat Parmesan, but don't overdo it.

Yogurt

You might be surprised to see yogurt listed as a carbohydrate on the *Buff Dad* chart because it's dairy, but on this plan it's considered a carb and not a protein like cottage cheese. Because it's a carb, you need to eat it with a protein just like you did with the pasta to make it a complete meal. Simply add half a handful of nuts to your yogurt, or eat it with an apple smeared with a spoonful of low-fat peanut butter.

Eat often: Low-fat plain or fruit yogurts, yogurt combined with cottage cheese.

Avoid: Frozen yogurt that is high in sugar and yogurts with more than 120 calories per serving.

Fruit

Just like yogurt and pasta, fruit needs to be combined with a protein to be considered a meal or snack. Dipping an apple in a spoonful of low-fat peanut butter or adding the fruit to low-fat cottage cheese are two easy ways to add protein. While adding sugary fruits such as canned peaches, pie fillings, or any type of processed fruits to cottage cheese are a *Buff Dad* no-no, adding fresh fruits including apples, pears, and cherries are perfectly fine and fit into the *Buff Dad* Dietary Plan.

The great thing about most fruits is they are portable and you don't need to measure them. One apple or one banana equals one serving, while it takes a cup of cut-up melon or berries to make a serving. They also don't need to be cooked, so they are perfect for on-the-go dads like you and me.

Eat often: All fresh fruits.

Avoid: Dried fruits such as those found in trail mixes, pie fillings, applesauces filled with sugar. Also avoid fruitlike processed snacks such as Fruit Roll-Ups.

Whole-Wheat Bread

Like pasta, even though bread is on the *Buff Dad* list, you've got to be careful of how much you eat and the types you eat. Check the package and look for breads with high fiber, at least 2 grams per serving, which keep you satisfied longer and are more useful for your body. I cannot stress the importance of not getting out of control. It's easy to go overboard when it comes to bread.

A serving of bread is either two slices of high-fiber bread or one tortilla, so if you're eating out, be careful. Those all-you-can-eat breadsticks at Olive Garden can be deadly to your buff dad waistline.

Eat often: Whole-wheat bread, tortillas, and pita breads.

Avoid: White breads, garlic toast, and pizza breads.

Vegetables

Filled with vitamins and nutrients not found in proteins or carbohydrates, vegetables are essential to your health. While you don't need to consume them at every meal, I do suggest at least two servings a day. Again, a serving is about the size of your fist or about a cup. Vegetables are also low in calories and high in fiber so they help move food through your digestive tract.

Eat often: Fresh and steamed vegetables. You can use light or balsamic vinegar to flavor salads (keeping the amount of dressing limited to a tablespoon). To add flavor to vegetables, cook them with dill, onion, or garlic. You can also add chili peppers, red peppers, or jalapeños for an extra kick.

Avoid: Fried, cheese-covered, or batter-coated varieties. Also avoid creamy salad dressings such as ranch and Caesar.

The Truth About Fats

I'm sure you've heard the saying "fat makes you fat." Well, I've got news for you. The people who say that are wrong—unless, of course, you're eating too much of it.

First of all, fat is needed for testosterone production. Without it, no matter how many vegetables and healthy high-fiber carbohydrates you're eating, you won't increase testosterone, which is the whole point of the program. Even if all you ate were the ten Big T power-foods, your body would still need fat to transform them into testosterone. Your body is like a sports car: you can fill it up with gas, but you need the key before you can put it in gear. Fat is your body's key.

Second, fat can readily be used for energy, providing you don't over-consume. Fat also stays in your stomach longer than protein and carbohydrates, making you feel full longer. Plus, fat tastes good, so it helps to eliminate cravings.

Daily Fat Consumption

Each day, the total number of fat grams you should consume is your body weight in pounds x .20. So, if you weigh 200 pounds, you should consume 40 grams of fat each day (200 x .20).

Feeding Your Fat Tooth

There are good fats and bad fats. The worst fats are the trans fats, which are mostly found in fast-food muffins, cookies, doughnuts, and deep-fried foods. Trans fats will not only make you fat, but they have been proven to cause heart disease. In fact, some cities in California and New York City have banned the use of trans fat all together. Other bad fats are the ones that are solid at room temperature, such as butter, margarine, and shortening.

Good fats include those found in liquid form as well as the essential fats found in fish and lean meats. So what happens if you don't eat these good fats? Well, you're not going to die, but you will feel a little under the weather. Symptoms of good fat deficiency include dry skin, a depressed metabolism, moodiness, decreased energy, dizziness, and even energy loss. Some of you may even be experiencing some of these problems now, as you don't have to be underweight to be undernourished. In fact, research shows that more than 95 percent of Americans don't eat enough good fats and are experiencing some of these symptoms.

Eat often: Good fats that are liquid, such as olive oil, canola oil, safflower oil, and sesame oil. Use flaxseed oil for uncooked items like salad dressings and in smoothies.

Avoid: Trans fats, solid fats like butter and margarine, and palm oil.

The Beer-Belly Blues

While the *Buff Dad* Dietary Plan lets you eat pretty much anything as long as you watch your serving sizes, one thing is not part of the plan: alcohol.

Yes, it's sad to say but there is a reason that beer-guzzling men don't have the bodies that aspiring buff dads like us want. According to research, the more alcohol you drink, the bigger waist-to-hip ratio you'll have. In other words, your waist will be larger than your hips.

A number of reasons account for this. First, alcohol causes your body to store fat in your belly area. But the second reason is even more devastating. Research shows that alcohol might not make you fatter on the scale, but it does diminish muscles in the gluteal and thigh regions. So you'll not only end up with a flabby tummy, but with skinny legs and a scrawny butt. I don't know about your spouse, but mine was not happy about this predicament at all. Apparently, she doesn't find that body type sexy. Go figure.

But don't worry. Staying away from the brew is only temporary. In twenty-eight days, you can have a nice cold one and toast your new buff body. Just don't make it a daily habit, or all your work will disappear.

Drink Water and Be Buff

The human body is made up of 60 percent water, but surprisingly your muscles are 80 percent water. So what happens if you don't drink enough water? Fortunately, your muscles won't deflate and turn your arms into sagging, prunelike appendages, but you will feel tired and irritable, and then your exercise will suffer due to fatigue.

But feeling a little run-down and exhausted is only the beginning. If you still don't fill up on water, your body will need to put extra energy into keeping you going. Your body will then be overworking, and you'll pay for it in other ways, such as stressing out your immune system. You may weigh 1 pound less on the scale, but you'll be more susceptible to colds, flus, and other viruses.

BUFF FACT

Keeping your body hydrated will help increase endurance, strength, and muscle fullness (how pumped out your muscles are), and speed up your metabolism.

In addition to keeping you healthy and happy, drinking water also helps reduce bloating and puffiness. I know it doesn't make sense, but remember how the body goes into starvation mode and stores extra fat when you diet? The same thing happens with water. When you don't drink enough, you'll look tired and puffy. But when you do drink enough, you'll look more toned because the body won't keep anything extra.

Unless you are drinking at least 64 ounces of water a day, you are not drinking enough. An easy way to tell if you're getting enough water is that your urine will be clear and odorless, unless of course you've just eaten asparagus or a bunch of beets. Another way to tell how much water you need is to weigh yourself before and after a workout. The difference between your pre- and post-workout weight is the average amount of water (or sweat) you lose during your training sessions. Each pound is approximately 16 ounces of fluid. To make sure you are drinking enough, aim for 64 to 128 ounces of water a day.

CHAPTER 6

THE *BUFF DAD* DIETARY PLAN

The Quick and Easy Way to Buffness

I'm a slow walker, but I never walk back.

Abraham Lincoln

It's easy to say you're going to lose weight. The hard part is actually doing it. As a former fat dad, I can completely attest to this fact. I've not only been on a number of diet and workout programs since I gained weight, but I've failed on every single one of them, except the *Buff Dad* program.

Almost every Monday morning, I'd start something new. The only problem was that I never actually stayed on any of the programs, which drove my wife crazy. It wasn't the diets that were annoying, but the process I'd go through. I'd tell myself (and her, as she's the only one willing to listen to me when I go off on these extreme diet rants) that I'm starting this new path of fitness and health. I would then begin cleansing the house of junk food—mostly by eating it. I'd then run out to the grocery store, buy a whole bunch of lettuce or whatever the latest diet told me to do, and tell my wife not to bother to tempt me. I was about to be transformed into a man of steel determination, even though I had a gut of blubber.

By the weekend, I'd have fallen off the diet wagon and restocked all the chips and soda. Needless to say, I was caught in a revolving door of doom and growing fatter by the week.

While part of the reason I failed on my many diet encounters may have been my own lack of dedication, other key elements played a role. The biggest one of these was hunger. I knew logically that I had enough fat stored in my body to live for weeks, but the body is a strange machine that doesn't always agree with logic. For example, why can't the body just transform jelly doughnuts into muscle? A calorie is a calorie, right? Unfortunately, the body doesn't work that way.

I'm sure many of you can remember back to the days when you could eat whatever you wanted and it magically burned away. Yes, those were the good days when the occasional binge wouldn't break the scale in the morning. The sad news is that sometime after the age of twenty-five, the body starts to slow down, and the instant calorie burning you experienced in your teens has now evolved into degeneration. In other words, instead of spending its energy rebuilding cells, the body starts to die, and you end up losing muscle, slowing your metabolism, and gaining weight.

Sounds depressing, doesn't it? The secret to preventing this from happening is to provide the body with food it can use. If the body can't use jelly doughnuts and deep-fried onion rings for energy and muscle building, it might be a good idea not to eat them, as they only end up turning into fat.

In a way, food is like impulse buying. Like many of you, I don't like to shop, but I do like to watch TV. I remember once I was flipping through the stations late on a Sunday night. My wife was already asleep upstairs with our son, and I was enjoying a relaxing moment of R&R when I came across this infomercial showing a cappuccino machine.

This wasn't just any old coffeemaker. This was a super-duper brewer that dripped your coffee like the professionals of Italy. At least that's what the guy said during the thirty-minute commercial. I couldn't resist. One phone call and two hundred dollars later, I was the proud owner of the Barista 2000. I unwrapped it, placed its heavy stainless-steel body on the counter, and then made myself a cup of coffee.

Unfortunately, that was the only cup I ever made. The Barista 2000 has now been sitting for the last six months on my counter, taking up space, which is exactly what unhealthy food does in your body. It might taste good and it's definitely tempting, but you don't really need it, and it ends up taking up precious space in your body in the form of fat.

Why the *Buff Dad* Dietary Plan Is Not a Diet

When designing the *Buff Dad* Dietary Plan, I wanted to make it as flexible as possible, and I wanted to make sure it didn't feel like a diet. If you're going to be buff, you might as well be buff for life. The way I see it, you should start eating like a buff dad right from the beginning rather than starving yourself on some sort of 400-calorie-a-day diet.

The "How" and "What" of Eating

Being lean and fit isn't rocket science. You don't need to have a die-titian, read a ton of books, or spend hours a day trying to figure out what to eat. The secret is eating the right amount of the right foods.

Let's start by figuring out how much you should eat. The *Buff Dad* program is all about portion control, but what exactly is a portion? A simple way to figure out how much food to put on your plate is to make a fist. If the amount of food is equal to the size of your fist, then you've got yourself a portion. For example, you'll want a fist's worth of pasta, another fist of vegetables, and a fist of protein.

Another way to estimate a serving size is to compare a piece of chicken or slab of meat to the palm of your hand. If it roughly is the same size, then that's the amount you're allowed to eat. Keep in mind it's only your palm. Fingers and wrists are not included.

Nothing is restricted on the *Buff Dad* Dietary Plan, because your body needs a little bit of everything in order to run efficiently. Cutting out one food group could leave you deficient, bloated, constipated, or run-down.

The *Buff Dad* Four-Week Action Plan

Every guy is different. Some of you like to create your own menus. Others like to mix and match. But for those of you who like to have everything all laid out, I've developed a four-week action plan to tell you exactly what you need to eat and how much. I've even included a weekly grocery list so you'll know exactly what to buy when you go shopping.

Even though I've laid it all out, there is still room for flexibility. You have three choices:

1   Plan your own meals by using the food chart provided in Chapter 4 and choosing foods from each of the three columns.

2   Modify existing recipes by substituting the regular ingredients with the *Buff Dad*–approved proteins and carbohydrates found on the testosterone list. For example, switch to lean ground turkey instead of hamburger and choose leaner cuts of meat.

3   If you were never big on cooking, you can use some of the recipes I've included.

Each of the thirty-four recipes is easy to prepare, takes little time, and doesn't include any fancy or unusual ingredients. In fact, most of the stuff you probably have in your refrigerator already. Also, because they don't take long to make, these recipes are easily whipped up after work. Others, like the Hearty Beef Stew, can even be prepared on the weekend and kept for quick and easy weekday meals or to-go lunches that can be microwaved at work.

The other good news is the *Buff Dad* Dietary Plan is designed for family dining. You (or your spouse) do not have to plan separate meals. All the recipes included in this book take into account the nutritional needs of your entire family. A side benefit is that you'll be less tempted because there's not going to be bad food left over in the fridge, nor will the rest of the family be eating pizza while you're suffering with a salad and protein drink.

Deep Down, We're All Cheaters

It's always nice to get a little something for nothing—whether it's finding an extra twenty dollars in a jacket pocket, coming to work and learning you've just received a raise without asking for it, or finding that parking place right in front of the mall door. The little rewards make your day worthwhile.

The problem I've found when dieting is that all my rewards are gone. Sure, I'm going to lose weight and look good if I stick to the regimented plan, but that's not going to satisfy me when I'm craving something I can't have. What will satisfy me is a greasy fast-food burger and a large order of fries.

In order to fix this problem and make the *Buff Dad* program work, I decided I needed to bend the rules a little. So I came up with three approved ways that you can cheat on the program and still lose weight.

You might be thinking you won't need to cheat. You're going to be one of those Mr. Dedication guys who can fight off all temptation to become a lean, mean buff dad machine. Well, if you can do this, then good for you. But I recommend taking advantage of the tips, because what's the point of being buff if you can't enjoy life and eat some of the good things that are available?

Besides, the *Buff Dad* program is not a temporary diet, but a new way of eating that you'll use for the rest of your life. Are you really ready to say good-bye to pepperoni pizza forever? Or are you ready to cheat a little and still get all the buff dad advantages while doing so? If the answer is "yes," read on and follow the rules.

Buff Rule #1: The *Buff Dad* 180-Minute Advantage

One of the problems with diets is that you're hungry all the time. Like you, I hate being hungry. The simplest solution to this problem is to eat. That's right. You don't need a doctorate in nutrition to figure out that once you eat, the hunger pangs magically disappear.

While you're on the *Buff Dad* program, you have my complete permission to eat every 180 minutes (or every three hours). I'm not saying you need to consume a whole chicken or slave over a hot stove for every meal. Instead, eat a little less than you would at a normal meal, but spread it out throughout the day.

And don't just eat a few celery sticks. That's not going to cut it. If you're going to eat, you should eat foods that are satisfying. By "satisfying" I don't mean go out to the local bakery and get a cream-filled pastry. Because the *Buff Dad* program is all about maximizing your time and energy, you should choose foods for your snacks that are going to build muscle and help increase your metabolism. So if you're going to eat all the time, you might as well lose weight and increase your testosterone as you do it.

To get the most out of your every-three-hour meals and to make sure you're never hungry, use the food chart provided in Chapter 4 and choose food combinations from each of the columns. Perhaps a scoop of cottage cheese with fresh fruit (remember no pie fillings or sugary canned fruits), grilled chicken with veggies in a whole-wheat pita pocket, or tuna salad on top of mixed lettuce greens will do the trick. It doesn't matter what you eat as long as you're eating every 180 minutes and it's on the list. Of course, just because you get to eat every three hours, it doesn't mean you can eat as much as your stomach can hold. Keep everything scaled down to a single serving.

Eating every 180 minutes not only gives you permission to cheat all day long, but it will also help you stay on the program. You'll never be hungry or feel starved because your body is always busy digesting the meal you just consumed.

Remember

A serving size is approximately that amount of food that could fit in the palm of your hand or the size of a clenched fist.

Buff Rule #2:
Eat One Free Meal a Week

In order to get the best results from the *Buff Dad* program, you're going to have to follow the workout program and dietary plan closely, but we can't be perfect all the time. One meal a week, I give you permission to eat whatever you want . . . and I mean *anything*. If you want a juicy burger piled high with a side order of cheese fries, go for it. If you want to eat a banana split and chocolate milkshake, do it. If you'd rather splurge and have pizza with real Coke, I don't mind. For one meal a week, you're allowed to go all out and be bad.

It doesn't matter what day you do it. Some people like to save their free meal for the weekend, but you can do it anytime you want. If you have an office party coming up, use your free meal then. Maybe you just had a really bad day and need to wallow in comfort foods, so you choose to have your freebie meal in the middle of the week.

Whether you use it as a treat or as an emergency binge to keep you going is up to you. Either way, just knowing that you can have your favorite foods once a week is going to keep you on the *Buff Dad* program for the long haul.

Believe it or not, having the chance to pig out once a week does more than help you get over your cravings for high-fat foods. It also helps convince your body you're not on a diet. That way, your body won't go into starvation mode and won't hold on to your fat. Pigging out can actually help you lose weight.

The other advantage of the free meal is that you will never feel deprived on the *Buff Dad* program because you know you can eventually have the stuff you like. It's much easier to make the *Buff Dad* program a lifestyle if you know you can eat what you want at least one meal a week.

The one final advantage of accepting that you're going to cheat once a week is that you won't be setting yourself up for disappointment. Remember how I said I would binge before every diet? One of the reasons was to prepare myself to never eat "bad" foods again.

No matter how keen you are in becoming the buffest dad in the universe, just saying you will never eat pizza or ice cream ever again is setting yourself up for failure. No one can be perfect. Even Brad Pitt and Mark Wahlberg have their off days. They may buff up for the camera, but I'm sure there are days when they relax with a beer and a pile of nachos smothered in salsa and cheese. Basically, cheating is going to help you in the long run. Just accept the fact that you're human and that high-fat food tastes good. Besides, knowing you can binge one meal a week will make the next week's workout and meal planning easier.

I should mention one other thing about the free meal. Sometimes it won't taste as good as you imagined. As your body gets used to eating foods that make it work more efficiently and you get used to having more energy, more strength, and more testosterone, you may find after eating a grease-filled meal that you feel sluggish and bloated. Don't worry. Your body just becomes used to digesting good foods during the week, so when you fill your body full of junk, you'll actually feel the difference. And the good news is, if you *do* feel a difference, you'll know you're on the right track.

Buff Rule #3:
Getting More Bang from Your Meals

This *Buff Dad* rule is not as fun as the other two, but kind of works along with them. So far, I've told you to eat every 180 minutes and to pig out once a week. But there are other ways to cheat to help the plan work faster and to make you feel full longer.

Here's a list of things I do to make the diet not a diet.

Never Drink Real Drinks

There is a reason that you don't see juice, milk, and soda in any of the three *Buff Dad* dietary columns, including freshly squeezed orange juice, skim milk, and diet sodas. While beverages may have some nutrition, they don't fill you up because they are easy to digest and have little or no fiber. So rather than wasting calories on fruit juice, eat real fruit or low-fat cheese and drink water instead. You'll find you get to eat more, and you'll feel fuller longer. The only beverages I've included are homemade protein smoothies, as they include more fiber and protein than traditional store-bought or processed drinks.

No Eating Before Bedtime

No bedtime snacks or drinks up to two hours before you sleep. When you sleep, your body's metabolism slows down. In other words, food that isn't digested by the time you fall asleep doesn't get burned off. Instead, it turns into fat.

Eat Two-Thirds of Your Daily Food Early

This tip goes along with the above tip and not eating before bed. To get the most out of the *Buff Dad* program, get used to eating two-thirds of your daily food intake before you get home from work. If you work at home or long hours, eat two-thirds of your food before 5:00 PM.

Many of you fast during the day, either because you're too busy to eat or you're just not hungry. The problem is that when you get home, you're starving. You either end up eating stuff you shouldn't eat just because you're so hungry, or you end up eating and going straight to bed. Spread out your meals throughout the day so your stomach is continuously working and burning calories all day long.

Eat Breakfast

You heard it before and now you're going to hear it from me: breakfast is the most important meal of the day, and this doesn't mean a coffee and muffin. Starting your day off with healthy food means you're starting to burn more calories earlier. When you're sleeping, your body slows down and saves energy, kind of like a mini-hibernation. Not until you eat again does your body wake up and kick into fat-burning mode. To make sure your body stays in fat-burning mode, continue eating every 180 minutes after breakfast.

Make a Shopping List

Making a shopping list helps you out in two ways. First, it's much easier to make the foods listed in the *Buff Dad* Dietary Plan if you have them in your house. Second, if your kitchen is stocked with healthy foods, even if you are tempted, the only things you can eat are healthy. Think about it: a late-night binge could only consist of chicken breast, whole grains, and fruits.

Drink Like a Fish

Notice I say "drink like a fish" and not like a frat boy. Drinking at least 10 cups of water a day does more than just help curb your appetite. Water is literally the fountain of youth. It will help plump up your muscles, reduce circles under your eyes, and flush out any impurities in your body. Let's face it: you want to look lean and buff, not like wrinkled leather.

The *Buff Dad* Ten Rules to Success

1. Eat every 180 minutes or every three hours.
2. Eat a combination of protein and carbohydrates at every meal.
3. Don't consume processed beverages.
4. Drink lots of water.
5. Eat two-thirds of your calories before leaving work or before 5:00 PM.
6. Indulge in one free meal a week.
7. Shop with a grocery list.
8. Eat breakfast.
9. Stop eating two hours before you go to bed.
10. Follow the *Buff Dad* Workout Blitz.

Buff Dad Success Story

Name: Alan, Father of Four

Before: 220 pounds

After: 180 pounds

Duration on program: 12 weeks*

Alan never considered himself as having a weight problem. After four children and watching the number creep higher and higher on the scale, he had to admit his weight was out of control. But gaining weight wasn't Alan's only problem. With his demanding job, he barely had time to eat, let alone go to the gym.

"My day consisted of waking up, grabbing a cup of coffee with sugar and cream, and heading off to the office. Lunch was usually something I picked up at a drive-thru window, and because I was starving after skipping breakfast, I usually would pick the biggest value meal on the menu. My most common choices were either a large cheeseburger and fries and regular Coke or Taco Bell," says Alan.

Alan's high-fat value lunch might have been economical, but the 1,200 calories he consumed added up over the years. Dinner was also fast food or something his wife would prepare for the family, such as pasta or fish and chips. His calories at dinner usually totaled around 2,500.

"I would eat dinner, and then I would have dessert with the kids— cookies or a couple of candy bars," says Alan.

The calories from Alan's after-dinner snacks totaled around 1,000 calories. All together, his daily intake was around 5,000 calories.

"When I started the *Buff Dad* program, I wasn't exercising at all and was weighing in at 220 pounds—and at 5'7", I'm not that tall," says Alan.

After twelve weeks on the *Buff Dad* program, Alan dropped 40 pounds and now consumes around 2,200 calories a day. Because of his fast-paced lifestyle, Alan still eats fast food, but he's making smarter choices. Instead of Taco Bell, he's choosing lower-fat and lower-carb choices, such as a six-inch Subway turkey sandwich with baked potato chips and diet soda. Dinner is lower in carbs, and he usually makes one of the *Buff Dad* recipes. He still has dessert with the kids, but now it consists of portion-control snack-size cookies (one package only) and a whole piece of fruit.

"And after twenty years, I'm back to eating breakfast and feeling great," says Alan. "It's amazing how little changes can make a big change to your life."

* Results vary on the *Buff Dad* program. Average weight loss is between 1 to 4 pounds a week depending on how heavy you are when starting the program.

CHAPTER 7

THE *BUFF DAD* WORKOUT BLITZ

You must have long-range goals to keep you from being frustrated by short-range failures.

Charles C. Noble

Now that you've mastered the ins and outs of the eating program, it's time to get down to business and start building those buff dad muscles. Yes, even if you are following the dietary plan exactly, you still need to work out. You may lose pounds by cutting back on fries and pizza, but without challenging your muscles, you'll still be soft in the middle. Think back to high school and the guy who was president of the Math Club. He might have been thin, but the girls weren't exactly drooling over him. You want fat loss, not muscle loss, and the best way to lose fat is to build more muscle while you're exercising.

Everything you need to achieve a buff dad body is right here in this chapter. It all comes down to what I call "supersetting," and it can be done either at a gym or in the comfort of your living room.

When supersetting during the *Buff Dad* Workout, you don't need to work out your entire body in every session. The better news is that you only need to weight train three times a week. You will also need to do two exercises for each muscle group to make sure your muscles stay balanced and cover the full range of motion.

Before we begin, I just have one word of advice: don't overdo it by doing a week's worth of exercise in one day. Too much exercise causes your testosterone levels to deplete, so it's better to work out effectively for shorter periods rather than for hours at a time.

The Not-So-Free Dad Lifestyle

If you are like me, the two most common reasons that you're not going to a gym or working out are lack of time and lack of motivation. The *Buff Dad* Workout Blitz combats both these problems because it takes little time to do, it can be done anywhere, and due to the type of exercises and the intensity, it provides noticeable results within weeks—giving you the motivation you need to continue. Sound good? Then let's get ready to lose some fat.

The *Buff Dad* Supersetting Secret

Supersetting is what makes the *Buff Dad* Workout Blitz effective. It helps you build the most muscle in the shortest amount of time. Sure, you can go to a gym and spend two hours a day pumping iron, but who has time for that? Instead, you can get the same results through the *Buff Dad* supersetting combinations in as little as 30 minutes, three times a week. Plus, the bonus is that you can split the 30 minutes into two 15-minute micro-workouts if you are really under time constraints.

What is supersetting? The short answer is that it's an interval training program that provides short, intense workouts. The exercises are simple, don't require a lot of equipment, and are designed to make sure you stick with the program over the long haul.

But the real secret behind supersetting is *how* you do the exercises. Normally when you lift weights, you do one set, wait 60 seconds, and do the next set. The problem is that during the waiting period your muscles have time to relax and start to recover.

With supersetting, you eliminate the recovery period, which challenges your muscles to work twice as hard and creates a more intense workout. Each supersetting exercise is actually a combination of two exercises that pair together opposing muscle groups. When you do both exercises—one after the other and no resting in between—it not only saves time by cutting out the rest period between sets, but because you're working opposing muscle groups (back and chest, biceps and triceps, hamstrings and quadriceps), you're increasing the intensity of the workout. The only rest the muscles get is while the opposite muscle is working.

In addition to saving time, there are even more benefits to this time-crunching madness. Working opposing muscles helps your body work together, which is actually better for your body than doing four different back exercises in one day and doing nothing for the chest muscles.

When working out one muscle group over and over, the opposing muscle overcompensates to fill in the fatigue. That's why you'll sometimes see people who work on the computer all the time walking slightly hunched or with rounded shoulders. Even though it doesn't feel like you're working out, the chest muscles are used in a lot of activities. Just sitting at a computer or driving keeps them activated at a low level all day. Even if you don't realize it, your chest muscles may be overdeveloped compared to your other muscles. And because you haven't worked out other parts of your body, the back muscles may not be strong enough to pull the chest back into alignment. The same thing happens when you work only one muscle group instead of opposing groups.

While you may not notice any problems at the beginning, you could end up with muscle imbalances that could lead to injuries. Lower back pain, hamstring pulls, and neck strain could all be prevented by making sure the opposing muscle groups are working equally.

The other great advantage to supersetting is that it allows you to overload the muscles without using heavy weights. This approach is perfect if you are a dad who is planning to tone up at home. With the lesser weights, you won't need to have a spotter hanging out in your living room or to invest in an expensive universal machine.

But let's not forget about the testosterone. The bonus to working opposing muscle groups is that the more muscles you involve in a workout, the more hormones are released. As a result, you'll be stimulating muscle growth all day long and not just during your session. In fact, your testosterone spikes when you work a lot of muscles at once such as with squats, dead lifts, and bench presses.

You've Got to Add Some Cardio

Just because you are pumping iron three days a week, don't think you're getting off easy on the other days. To get the full benefit of the *Buff Dad* Workout Blitz, you are going to have to do some cardio.

Yes, that means breaking a sweat and raising your heart rate high enough so that you can burn off enough fat and actually see the muscles you are building.

The good news is, just like the muscle resistance training portion of the workout, you only need to do cardio three times a week and only for 30 minutes. The type of cardio you do is completely up to you. It could be jogging, biking, speed walking, swimming, or working out on a stair-climber or elliptical runner. You're free to choose your cardio exercise and go with it. You can also switch things up and do 15 minutes of biking and 15 minutes on the stair-climber. Basically, you can do anything you want as long as your heart rate rises and stays elevated for 30 minutes.

The one thing I will warn you about is doing too much. Believe it or not, overdoing your cardio can be a bad thing. Not only is it bad for your joints if you're running every day or doing excessive aerobic sessions, but too much can also cancel out your muscle gains.

My advice is to keep the cardio sessions to 30 to 45 minutes. There's no sense working out until exhaustion if it's not going to give you the results you want, but I do want you to sweat and sweat enough that on a scale of one to ten, you're clocking in at eight. If you're going to do the cardio, you might as well get the maximum benefits, which means doing more than a leisurely walk. A recent study from Duke University found that people who performed higher-intensity workouts were able to significantly lower their abdominal fat levels and lose weight relatively quickly. But those people who did low-intensity cardio such as walking for 30 minutes and not raising their heart rates didn't lose anything. In fact, on average they gained 1.5 pounds over the eight months of the study. I'm not saying walking isn't right for you. Depending on your fitness level, walking may raise your heart rate and cause you to sweat. I'm just saying, make the time you work out worth it—sweat it out and honestly be able to say you're working at 80 percent.

Now before you start cheating and think you are only going to do 20 minutes or 10 minutes of cardio, let me explain the reasoning behind the 30-minute plan. Research shows that 30 minutes of cardio is the optimal amount you need to lose weight and burn fat. When you do cardio, you burn fat up to 50 percent more effectively than you would performing low-intensity workouts such as weight training. Plus, you get the extra advantage of having your metabolism revved up for a few hours after you stop working out—which means you continue to burn excess calories even after you are done breaking a sweat.

BUFF FACT

A 2005 study in the *European Journal of Sports Science* reveals that just 15 minutes of cardio three times a week could drastically reduce

The Best Time to Burn Fat

Although not a necessity, the best time to do your cardio is first thing in the morning before you eat your breakfast. Studies indicate that fat is burned three hundred times faster during morning exercise compared to evening or afternoon workouts. A study performed at Kansas State University revealed that a kilogram of fat is burned sooner when exercise is done in the fasted state in the morning than when done later in the day. The reason is that early in the morning, your levels of glycogen (which is what your body turns carbohydrates into) are low.

While you are sleeping, your levels of glycogen slowly decline. Carbs (or glycogen) are your body's primary and preferred energy source. When your primary fuel source is in short supply, your body taps into its reserve energy source: body fat. Basically, working out in the morning forces your body to burn more fat because it has no other fuel to use.

Of course, if you work out at any other time of the day, you'll still burn fat; you'll just burn less of it because you'll first be burning off the carbohydrates you ate. But really what's most important is not *when* you work out, but *that* you work out.

How to Do Your Cardio

You should perform your cardio as if you're running up a mountain. Start off slow and increase to medium intensity. Once you're about 12 to 15 minutes into your workout, increase your intensity level to high for about 7 to 10 minutes, and then start bringing it back down so that you end your last few minutes back where you started.

While you are working for a good half hour, you are really only pushing yourself to the edge for 10 minutes of the total workout. The rest of the time is spent building up to that peak and slowing back down.

Of course, as your fitness level improves, so will your intensity. You'll have to run faster, tighten the exercise bike tension more, or start walking uphill. The last thing you want to do is plateau in your cardio. If you're not sweating, you're not burning fat.

To summarize, for the optimal results from the *Buff Dad* Workout Blitz, you need to lift weights three times a week for 30 minutes and then do some sort of cardio exercise three times a week for 30 minutes.

The *Buff Dad* Workout Blitz by Week

One of the great things about the *Buff Dad* Workout Blitz is that you'll be working your entire body in each 30-minute session. In order to cut back on time, some workout programs split the body in half and train half the muscles on one day and the other half on the other. Because of the supersetting technique, the *Buff Dad* Workout Blitz is designed to ensure you work out all of your muscle groups every time—giving you twice the benefits in the same amount of time. Plus, as supersetting eliminates the rest period between the sets, you can do more exercises in a 30-minute time period while effectively fatiguing your muscles.

 WEEK 1

Monday	Total body (quads, hamstrings, chest, shoulders, back, biceps, triceps, and abs)
Tuesday	30 minutes of aerobic exercise
Wednesday	Total body (quads, hamstrings, chest, shoulders, back, biceps, triceps, and abs)

Thursday   30 minutes of aerobic exercise

Friday   Total body (quads, hamstrings, chest, shoulders, back,
              biceps, triceps, and abs)

Saturday   30 minutes of aerobic exercise

Sunday   Rest

 WEEKS 2–4: REPEAT WEEK 1.

While you'll be repeating the same training schedule each week during the four-week program, *how* you'll actually be lifting will vary. Some days you'll be lifting lighter weights and doing more repetitions, and other days you'll be lifting heavier weights, but doing less reps. The reason for the change is to trick your muscles into working hard each and every time. Plus changing up the quantity and volume will help prevent fitness plateaus and keep your body working toward looking buff and lean.

Later in the book, I show you step-by-step how to do the exercises to work each muscle group effectively.

Squeezing in the Thirty Minutes

Even if you have the tightest of schedules, squeezing an extra 30 minutes into your day is possible. However, if you are not sure how to get a little more out of your day, here are a few tips:

Split the weight-training segment up into two 15-minute programs. Do chest, shoulders, and back in the morning before work, and then quads, hamstrings, biceps, triceps, and abs after work.

Find a way to do your cardio during your lunch hour—anything from a brisk walk around the building, keeping your bike in the back of the minivan and going for a quick ride, or running up and down stairs for 30 minutes.

If working out at home is impossible, consider joining a gym. While the program is designed to be done at home for optimal convenience, it also can be done at a fitness center. With a gym membership, you have the flexibility of going into work 30 minutes earlier for a quick workout before the start of your day, working out at lunchtime, or squeezing in a quick 30-minute cardio session after work.

CHAPTER 8

KEEPING THOSE MUSCLES GROWING

Winners never quit and quitters never win.

Ted Turner

I f you've worked out before, you know that hitting the dreaded plateau is always a problem. For those of you who have never been to a gym or haven't gone consistently, what happens is that when you first start working out, you'll see results, but after a while your muscles get used to the intensity and it no longer becomes work. Some of you might even experience an initial weight gain as you start lifting weights. This is because muscle weighs more than fat. So while you may be losing inches, the scale might not actually reflect your results. If this is the case, don't be discouraged. Keep on with the program and as the muscles you build start burning calories, you'll shed those fat dad pounds. But if you hit a plateau, then it's a whole different story.

What happens when you hit a fitness plateau is that instead of rebuilding after each workout, the muscles settle into a routine, kind of like you did after becoming a dad, and while you continue to spend the same amount of time working out, you'll no longer see continued results. This is why you'll see some guys going to the gym every day and never looking any better.

Because they aren't stimulating their muscles in new ways, they are stuck in the same place—even though they are still working out every day and lifting the same amount of weight they did a couple of months ago. In fact, if these poor guys continue following their status quo, their muscles will be so efficient at doing the workout that they are actually going to start losing tone.

I don't know about you, but for me, this is really discouraging, especially if I'm putting in precious time to look buff. But I do have good news. To combat this problem, I've developed a solution that tricks the muscles into not falling into a routine. It all has to do with the number of reps you do with each exercise and how much weight you're lifting.

Normally, when you work out you do 8 to 12 repetitions (reps) of the exercise while lifting as much as you can. You then rest and repeat the exercise until you've done the same thing three times in a row. You do the exact same routine the next time you work out.

That's where the problem occurs. Because you're doing the same thing each time you work out, there's more chance your muscles are going to remember the pattern and plateau. With the *Buff Dad* Workout Blitz, this won't happen. The secret is simple: you vary the pattern, following my guidelines, of course.

Remember how I mentioned that you'll be doing the same workout every week, but *how* your workout would change? This is where the change comes in and why it's important to follow the program exactly. In the *Buff Dad* Workout Blitz, you'll be supersetting your exercises (working opposing muscles) and eliminating any rest periods in between. This alone starts to fatigue the muscles and reduces plateaus, but to get ultimate *Buff Dad* results, you'll need to change up the number of reps you do and the amount of weight you lift to continuously challenge your muscles. This will ensure you get the most out of your workout each and every time. Failing to impose new challenges such as increasing how much you lift will keep you at the same size rather than spur new muscle growth.

To get the maximum results for each exercise, you'll have to use weights heavy enough that your muscle feels fatigued on the final repetition. You'll also be doing three sets of each exercise.

The Perfect Team to Make You Lean

Many of you are probably thinking, *Okay, this supersetting stuff makes sense. What if I only do this and not diet?* I hear you and, yes, you can do only the workout portion and you will build muscle. You'll be bigger and stronger, but you'll still be fat. If you want to look good, you must do both the diet and the workout portions.

I've already mentioned I'm the lazy type. If there was an easier way, I would have found it. But this is how I see it: if I'm going to get out of bed and work out for 30 minutes every day, I want the world to see my results. It's not going to matter that you can lift an additional 20 pounds and do one hundred abdominal crunches if all your hard work is hidden beneath a layer of fat. If you're going to do the work, you might as well have the visual results to prove it.

The diet and workout program combine to get you the best results. The meal plan controls your weight and, through its low-fat, high-testosterone-building foods, helps you build muscle quickly. The workout portion utilizes these foods to help build the muscle and burn off the dad fat.

Toning Up at Home or in the Gym

Before I became a dad, I was a gym rat. I worked out religiously and had no problem getting myself to a gym. While my gym bag and running shoes are still in the back of the car, I haven't actually stepped inside the walls of the fitness club since the day my son was born. Sadly, I don't miss it.

Every man has his own way of working out. Some of you feel comfortable going to a fitness club, while others find it's more practical to work out in the comfort of your home. Where you work out doesn't matter, as long as you do it. Because of this, I've made sure that all the exercises in the *Buff Dad* Workout Blitz can be done in your living room, in a gym, or even on the road. If you don't want to take your free weights with you, you can easily do the workout in the hotel's fitness room.

Don't worry. You won't need to transform your home into a heavy-duty sports club. All you're going to need is some free weights and a stability ball or a chair. If you do decide to use a stability ball (these are the big blow-up balls you might have seen on TV or at the gym), look for one that matches your height by reading the size recommendations on the box. The balls come in different sizes—small, medium, and large. Pump it up so that it's large enough that when you sit on it, your knees are at a 90-degree angle. However, with the *Buff Dad* Workout Blitz, it's not the equipment that matters, but the supersetting technique and how the exercises are performed that are going to give you the toned look you want.

And no, you won't be doing girly aerobic moves or dancing along to a video. You'll be building muscle and pushing your body to the limit. You'll see results in as little as four weeks. All you have to do is follow along.

Buff Dad Success Story

Name: Greg, Father of Two

Before: 245 pounds

After: 180 pounds

Duration on program: 6 months*

Greg is 6'1" and a forty-year-old father of two. In his early thirties, he was already weighing in at over 200 pounds, but in the eight years after the birth of his kids, Greg's weight escalated.

"I gained an additional 25 pounds after the kids were born," says Greg. "I was at my heaviest, weighing in at 245."

Before starting the *Buff Dad* program, Greg was eating three meals a day; snacking on high-carb, high-fat, sugary foods; and drinking beer daily. He didn't have time for a regular exercise routine, and the only physical activity he did was playing the occasional basketball game or playing with the children at the park.

Greg works ten- to twelve-hour days, so time was a factor in getting buff. He usually ate on the run, in meetings, or in the car.

"Because of my long days, dinner was usually after 8:00 PM and was whatever my wife would make for the family," says Greg. "My favorite meal was pizza and beer."

After trying a couple of diets on his own and failing, Greg decided to get serious about his weight loss and try the *Buff Dad* program.

"I didn't think it would work for me," says Greg. "But after losing 65 pounds, I feel like a new man."

Greg dropped an amazing 65 pounds in six months and gained muscle mass. Now he weighs 180 pounds and feels like a twenty-year-old. In addition to looking good and feeling great, he has more energy and enjoys playing with his kids when he gets home from work or on the weekend.

* Results vary on the *Buff Dad* program. Average weight loss is between 1 to 4 pounds a week depending on how heavy you are when starting the program.

CHAPTER 9

FOUR WEEKS TO A
BUFF DAD

Putting the Plan into Action

Keep away from people who try to belittle your ambitions.
Small people always do that, but the really great make you
feel that you too can become great.

Mark Twain

It's time to get started! I know you're excited and want to dive right into the core of the workout, but I can't stress enough the importance of warming up before you work out and cooling down when you're done. This doesn't mean doing a couple of neck stretches or hopping in the shower when you're done. Instead, you need to warm up your muscles with real exercises.

Think of it this way: your muscles need a little pre-exercise to get prepared before you start doing the "real" workout. If you don't, they won't work properly, you won't be able to lift as much weight, and there's a chance you'll overstretch some tendons and cause pain. Basically, you won't be at your best during the workout.

What You'll Need

1 stability ball

Dumbbells: 10 pounds, 15 pounds, 20 pounds or resistance tubing

Bridge Chair or some no-arm chair

Warming Up

Your warm-up doesn't have to be anything fancy. If you're at home, I recommend jogging in place and swinging your arms for a couple of minutes or running up and down the stairs a couple of times, taking two stairs at a time. If you're at the gym, do a quick 5-minute cardio session on the treadmill, stationary bike, or elliptical runner. You don't have to go full steam, just enough to warm up your core temperature.

BUFF FACT

Water helps relieve muscle tension and soreness by flushing out the lactic acid that builds up during a workout. Drink plenty of it.

Building Muscles the *Buff Dad* Way: The *Buff Dad* Workout Blitz

In order to get buff on the program, you don't need any fancy equipment, but you do need to do the exercises at least three times a week. Here is an overview of all of the exercises in the Workout Blitz. Once you're familiar with these, you can customize your three-day-a-week strength-training sessions by working opposing muscles, or turn to the complete workout that begins on page 119.

One important rule to keep in mind is that even though you are supersetting the workout, you should not do the exercises superfast. Instead, in order to get the maximum benefits and to decrease your chance of injury, do each exercise slow and controlled. I recommend counting to four with each movement. In other words, when the exercise says to "slowly" squat down, your squat should take four counts to go down and four counts to come back up.

Dumbbell Squats

Stand, holding a pair of dumbbells, with your feet shoulder width apart and your knees unlocked. Bring the weights up in front of your body and rest the end of each dumbbell on the top of each shoulder— your palms should be facing each other with your elbows pointing out. Slowly squat down until your thighs are parallel to the floor. Pause, slowly push yourself back into a standing position, and repeat.

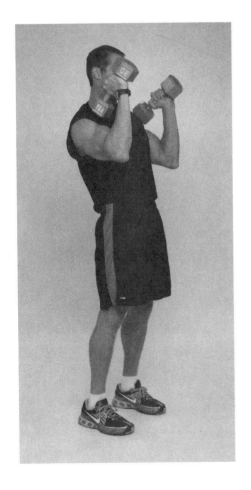
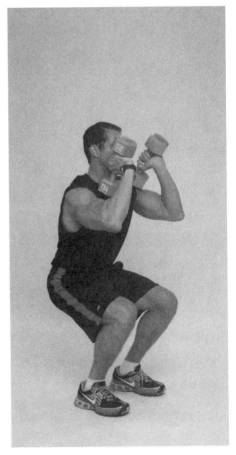

Dumbbell at Side Squats

Stand with your feet shoulder width apart and place the dumbbells just outside of each foot. Bend your knees and grab the dumbbells with your palms facing in toward your knees. Keeping your head up and your back straight, slowly stand up until your legs are straight but your knees aren't locked. Keep the weights close to your body as you lift. Pause, slowly lower the weights back down to the floor, and repeat.

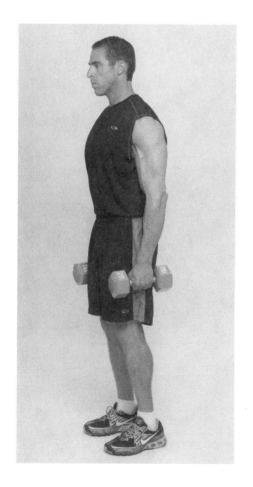 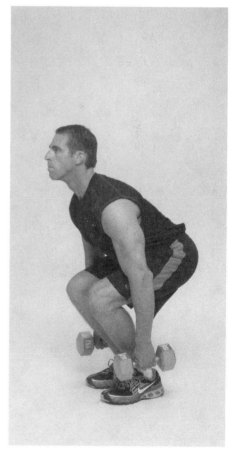

Bent-Over Rows

Stand straight with light dumbbells in each hand, arms down at your sides. Bend forward at the waist until your back is parallel to the floor. Your legs should be straight but unlocked; your arms should hang straight down with palms facing each other. While keeping your arms close to your torso, raise both dumbbells straight up until they touch the sides of your chest. Pause, slowly lower the weights until your arms are straight once more, and repeat.

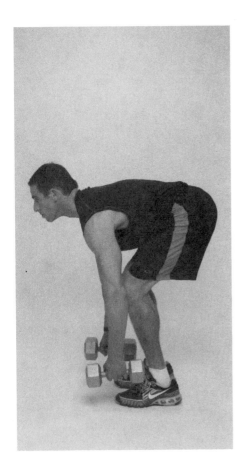
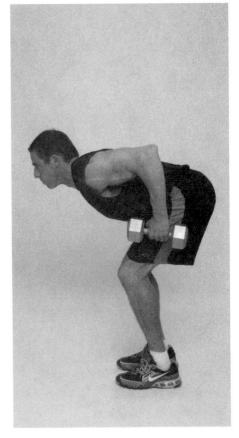

Stiff-Leg Deadlifts

Stand with your feet shoulder width apart and your knees unlocked. Bending only at your waist, grab the dumbbells so that your palms face in toward your feet. Keeping your back flat and your legs straight (knees slightly unlocked), slowly raise yourself back up into the standing position until the weights end up in front of your thighs. Do not pull with your arms; they should stay straight throughout the exercise, but not locked at the elbows. Pause, lower the weights back to the floor, and repeat.

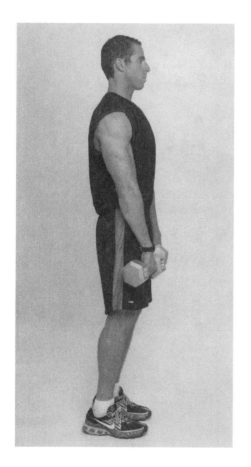 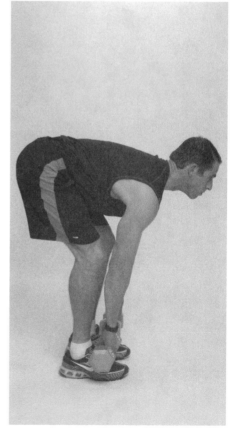

Lunges

Stand with dumbbells in each hand, palms facing in, your arms hanging at your sides, and your feet about shoulder width apart. Keeping your back straight, step forward with your right foot and lean forward until your right thigh is almost parallel to the floor. Gently push yourself back into the starting position and repeat, this time stepping out with your left foot and repeat.

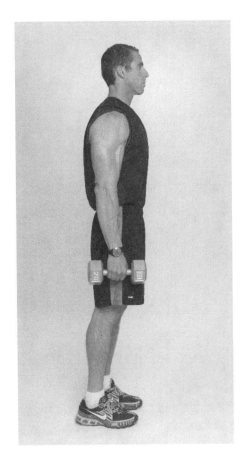 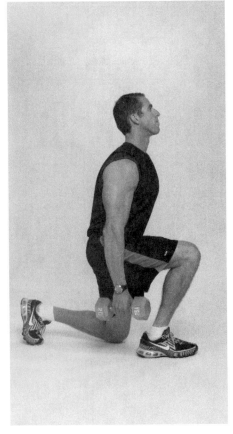

Side Lateral Raises

Stand straight with your feet shoulder width apart and hold light dumbbells in each hand. Your arms should hang down, and your palms should face in toward each other. Keeping your arms straight, slowly raise them out to your sides until they're parallel to the floor. (You'll look like the letter T.) Pause at the top of the movement for a second, then slowly lower your arms back down to your sides, and repeat.

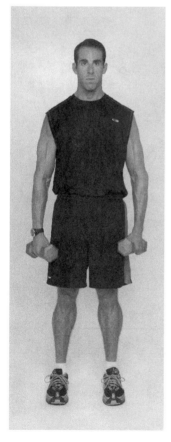
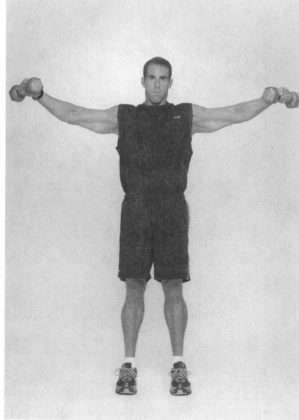

Biceps Curls

Stand holding dumbbells in each hand, with your arms hanging at your sides and your palms facing out in front of you. Keeping your back straight, slowly curl the weights up. Your palms should end up facing the fronts of your shoulders. Slowly lower the weights back down and repeat.

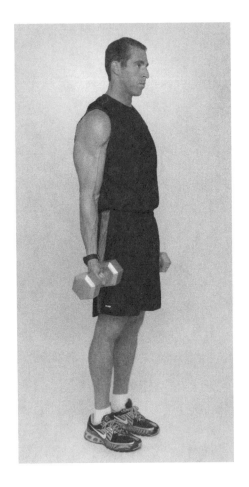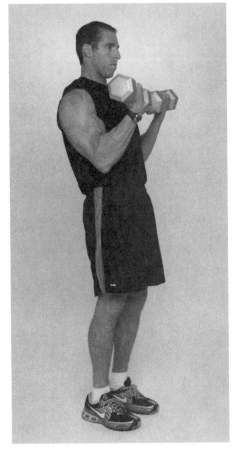

Push-Ups

Place your hands flat on the floor (shoulder width apart) with your arms straight and elbows unlocked. Straighten your legs behind you, drawing your feet together. Rise up on your toes so the top of the balls of your feet are touching the floor. Your body should be a straight line from your heels to your head, your eyes focused straight down at the ground. Without moving your head, slowly lower until your upper arms are parallel to the ground. Pause, slowly push yourself back up, and repeat.

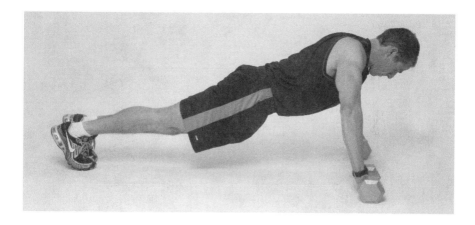

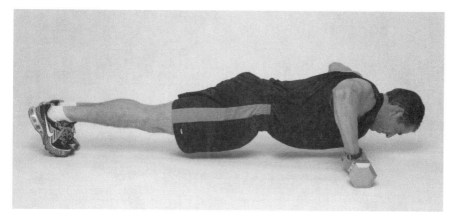

Biceps Concentration Curls

Sit on the edge of a chair with a light dumbbell in your right hand. Keeping your back straight, bend at the waist so that your right arm hangs down between your legs. The back of your right arm should rest on the inside of your right thigh, palm facing in. (Your left hand can rest on your left knee.) Keeping your upper arm pressed against your thigh, slowly curl the weight up to your right shoulder. Lower the weight back down until your arm hangs straight once again, and repeat. Afterward, switch positions to work with your left arm.

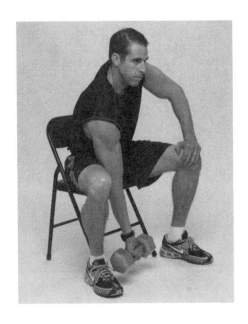 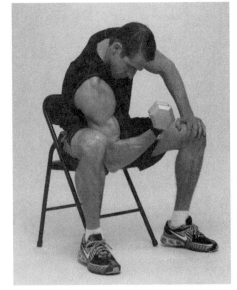

Triceps Extensions

Sit on the edge of an exercise bench, chair, or stability ball with a light dumbbell in your right hand. Raise the weight straight up over your head and rotate the dumbbells so that your right palm faces left. Press your right biceps against the side of your head, using your left hand to support your right elbow. Slowly lower the weight behind your head as far as you can, keeping your wrist straight throughout the exercise. Raise the weight overhead until your arm is straight. Repeat for one set, then switch hands to work with your left arm.

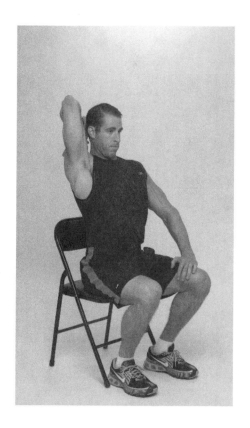 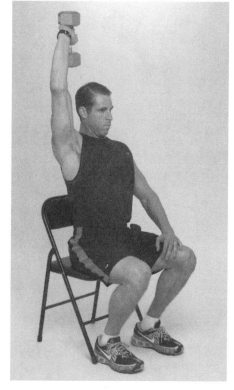

Dips

Sit on a sturdy chair and shuffle your butt forward, placing your palms on the chair with your fingers hanging off the front edge. Keeping your hands in place, slowly step forward until your feet are in front of you. You can do this exercise with your knees bent, but the straighter your legs are, the harder the exercise will be as your triceps will need to support more weight. Your arms should be straight with elbows unlocked, supporting your weight behind you. Slowly lower yourself until your butt is as close to the floor as possible without touching it. Press back up until your arms are straight, elbows unlocked, and repeat.

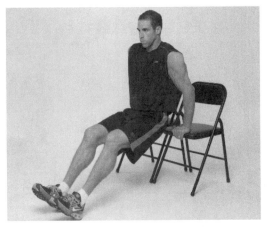

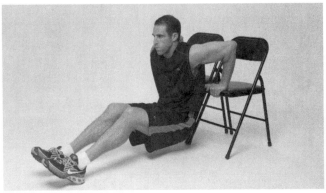

Shoulder Press on a Stability Ball

Sit down on a stability ball with a dumbbell in each hand. (You can also use a chair for this exercise.) To help maintain your balance, spread your feet slightly wider than shoulder width apart, keeping your feet flat on the floor. Bring the weights up to the sides of your shoulders, your palms facing forward. Keeping your back straight, slowly press the weights over your head until your arms are straight, elbows locked. Lower the weights back down to your shoulders and repeat.

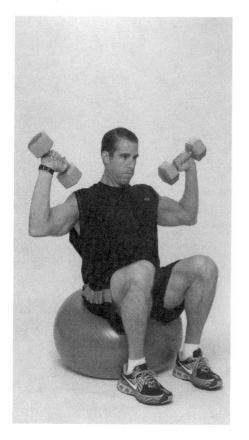 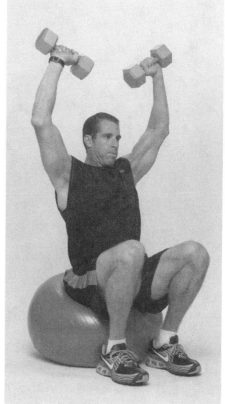

Crunches on a Stability Ball

Sit on top of a stability ball with your legs in front of you and your feet flat on the floor. Slowly lean back and roll yourself down the ball until just your head, shoulders, and back are touching it; your back should shape itself to the curve of the ball. Touch your hands lightly alongside your ears, and you're ready to begin. Keeping your balance, slowly lift your head, arms, and upper back off the ball. Lower back down and repeat. If you don't have a stability ball, lie down on the floor and do the exercise from there.

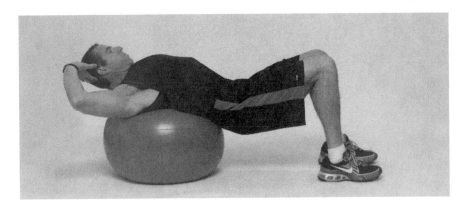

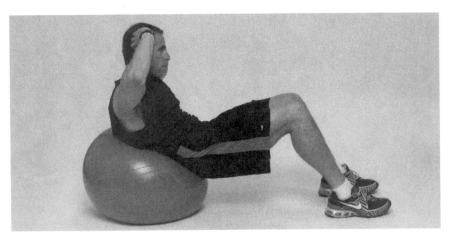

Reverse Crunches on a Stability Ball

Get on the floor as if you were about to perform a push-up, placing your hands shoulder width apart. But instead of straightening your legs with your feet on the floor, rest the front of your shins on a stability ball. With your arms straight and your back flat, your body should form a straight line from your shoulders to your ankles. Slowly roll the ball forward with your feet, toward your chest, raising your hips and rounding your back as you go. Pause, return to the starting position, and repeat. If you don't have a stability ball, lie on the floor

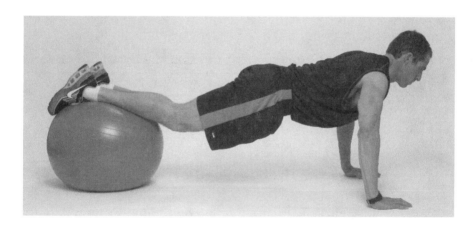

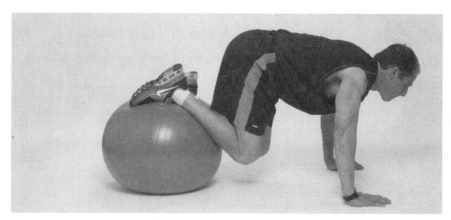

on your back with your legs stretched out in front of you. Slowly raise your legs to 90 degrees making sure you don't "swing" them up, but use your ab muscles. Pause, then slowly lower your legs down, being careful not to arch your back. Repeat.

Wall Squats Using a Stability Ball

Stand with your feet 18 to 24 inches apart with your lower back pressed firmly against a stability ball. Lean back against the ball on a sturdy wall, slowly bend your legs, and lower yourself down. Sliding against the ball until your thighs are parallel with the floor, pause, then push yourself back up into a standing position and repeat. If you don't have a stability ball, perform the exercise without the wall.

Biceps Curls on a Stability Ball

Grab two dumbbells with an underhand grip and sit on a stability ball or chair. Keeping your upper arms planted on the ball, curl the dumbbells up as high as you can. Resist the urge to lean back; you want your biceps to do all the work. Pause, slowly lower the dumbbells back down, and repeat.

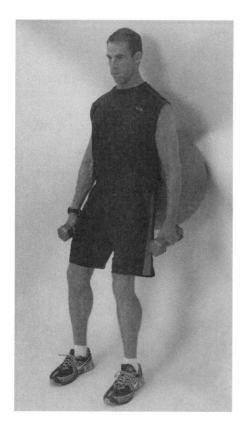

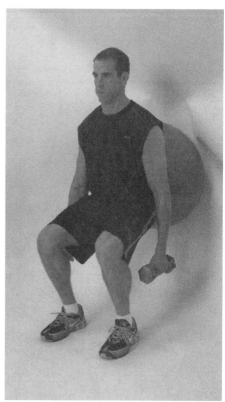

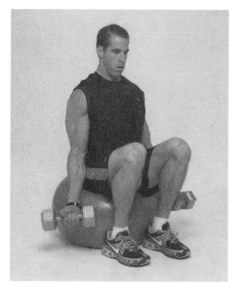

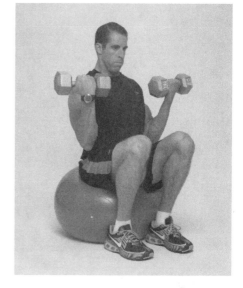

Incline Press on a Stability Ball

Lie back on a stability ball with a dumbbell in each hand. Raise the weights so that they rest along the outside of your chest, with your palms facing forward. Slowly press the dumbbells straight up above your chest, touching them together at the top. Avoid locking your elbows, which will take tension off your chest muscles. Slowly lower the weights back along the sides of your chest and repeat. You can lie back on the seat of a chair if you don't have a stability ball.

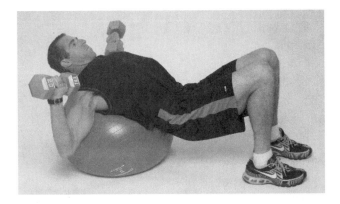

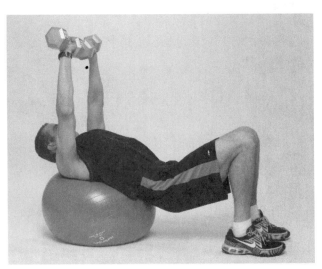

Buff Dad
Post-Workout Stretches

Your cooldown is just as important as your warm-up. The last thing you want to do after a good workout session is go right to sleep. Besides, stretching has been proven to speed up recovery and increase a muscle's range of motion, and more motion means there's more room for muscle fibers to grow.

Lying Glute Stretch

Lie on your back with both legs flat on the floor. Bend your right leg and place your right foot over your left leg, resting it flat on the floor on the outside of your left thigh. Grab below your right knee and gently pull it toward your chest as far as is comfortable, keeping your upper body flat on the floor, and hold for 10 seconds. Relax, repeat, then switch positions to stretch your left leg.

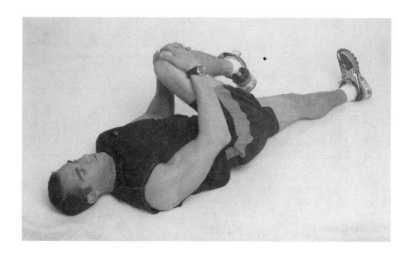

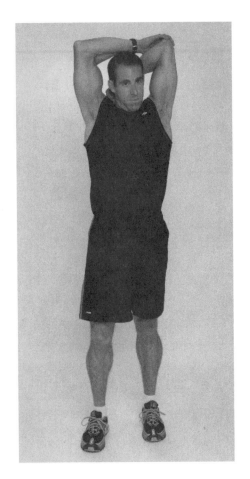 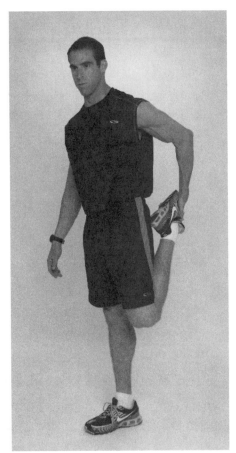

Triceps and Lats Stretch

Raise your right arm straight over your head, then bend it at the elbow so that your right hand drops behind your head, touching your neck. You should look as if you were about to stretch your upper back. Take your left hand, grab your right elbow with it, and gently push your right arm backward slightly for 10 seconds. Switch arms and repeat.

Standing Quadriceps Stretch

Stand on your left foot. Reach back with your right hand and grab your right ankle. Maintaining this position, gently push your hips forward, pull on your right ankle, and hold for 10 seconds. Relax, repeat once more, and then switch positions to stretch your left leg.

Lying Back Twist

Lie flat on your back with your legs straight and your arms down at your sides. Bend your left leg and plant your left foot flat on the floor next to your butt; your left knee should point to the ceiling. Reach across your body with your right hand and grab the outside of your left knee. Keeping your knee bent, gently pull your left leg over to your right side as you simultaneously twist your torso to the left. Hold for 10 seconds and then gently twist yourself back. Change positions—drawing your right knee up and keeping your left leg down—and repeat the stretch on that side.

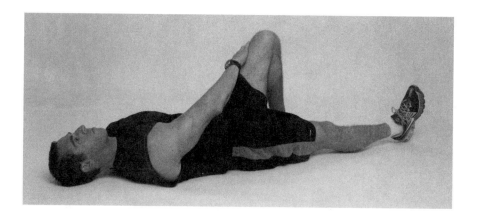

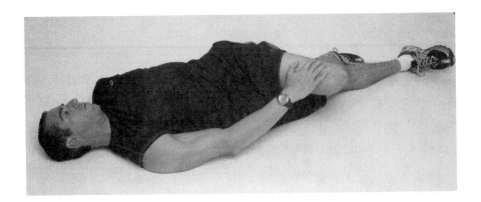

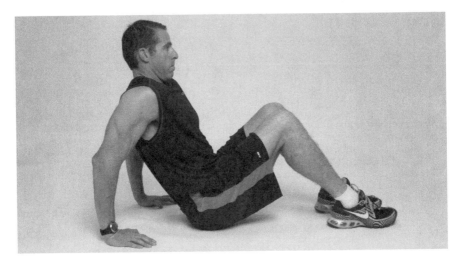

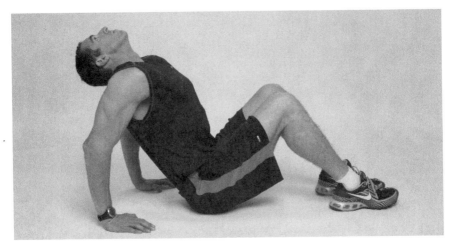

Arch Stretch

Sit down on the floor with your knees bent and your feet flat. Reach back as far as possible and place your hands behind you, your palms flat and your fingers pointing away from your body. Your feet should stay on the floor. Lift up your chest and arch your back so that you draw back. Tilt your head back, chest high up, and hold the position for 10 seconds. Relax and repeat the stretch again to loosen up.

Standing Bent-Over Hamstring Stretch

Stand with your feet shoulder width apart, straight ahead and a slight bend in your knees. Bend over at the waist and touch your toes with your fingers. Make sure your knees are slightly bent and hold for 10 seconds. Do not bounce. After the hold, slowly raise your upper body to the starting position and repeat.

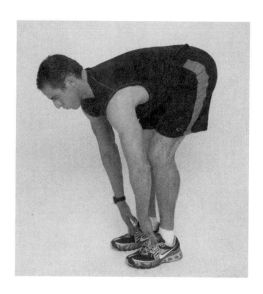

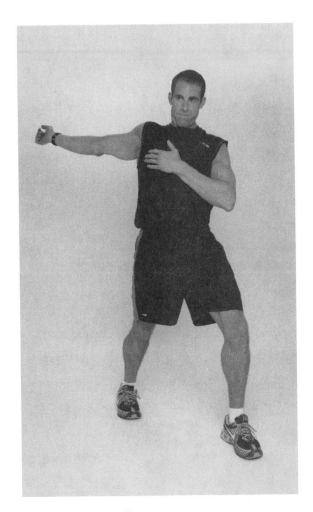

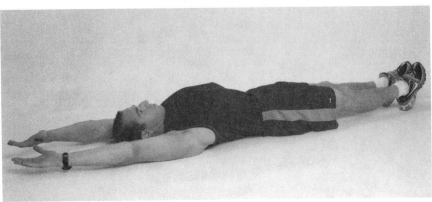

Standing Chest Stretch

Extend your right arm straight out away from your chest. Keep your right arm high and act like you are throwing a baseball. You should feel the stretch along your right chest and shoulder. Hold for 10 seconds, then switch positions and stretch your left. Repeat 2 stretches for each arm.

Stretch and Reach

Lie flat on your back with your arms directly overhead—your upper arms alongside your ears—your legs straight. Reach back with your fingers while pointing your toes. Imagine that you are being pulled apart. Breathe in your ab muscles and hold for 10 seconds. Slowly return to the starting position and repeat.

Shoulder Stretch

Extend your right arm straight across your chest as if you were reaching over to the left. Grab your left arm up and underneath your right arm, then use it to gently pull your right arm closer in toward your chest. You should feel the stretch along your right shoulder. Hold for 10 seconds, then switch positions to loosen your left shoulder.

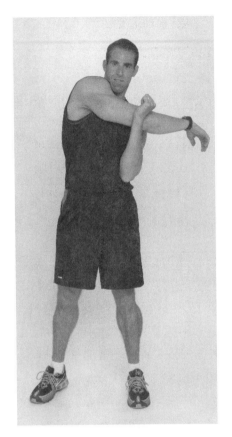
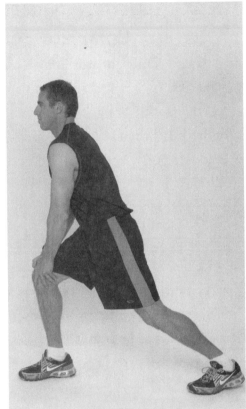

Standing Calf Stretch

Stand with your feet shoulder width apart and your toes pointing out in front of you, then step forward with your left foot. Place your hands on top of your left thigh, just above your knee, and gently straighten your right leg until your heel is flat on the floor. You should be straight, hips forward, with your head up as you hold the stretch for 10 seconds. Change positions and repeat with the other leg.

Buff Dad Three-Day-a-Week Complete Body Workout

I'm sure you've noticed that there are a number of exercises in the workout. The good news is you won't have to do every single one of them each time. You'll only have to do nine of them. Because some of the exercises work the same muscles, just in slightly different ways, the program mixes them up each day. This way your body is constantly challenged and is less likely to plateau.

Workout Overview

You will do each of the nine exercises continuously, stopping only if you need to catch your breath. Once you finish one set of all nine exercises, you go back to the beginning and do the sequence two more times, to make a total of three sets of each exercise, EXCEPT for the ab exercises, of which you only have to do two sets. Before you begin, consider these guidelines:

1 **Circuit train.** Do one set of all nine exercises one after another until you complete the full sequence. Do not rest in between unless you have to take a quick breather. Then go back to the first exercise and repeat the full sequence again. You'll go through the circuit three times.

2 **Rest 1 minute only after completing the entire sequence of exercises.** (Do not rest between exercises unless you absolutely have to.)

3 Increase the weights, decrease the reps. For best results, perform set #1 using dumbbells you can lift at least 15 times; for
most guys, this will be 10-pound dumbbells. On the second set,
increase your weight to 12-pound dumbbells and decrease the
number of reps to 12. For the third set, increase the weight again to
15-pound dumbbells and perform 10 reps. As you build muscle, you
can continue to increase the weight of the dumbbells.

Workout Circuit Day 1

DUMBBELL SQUATS

1 set of 15 reps with 10-pound dumbbells

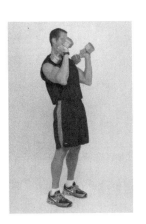 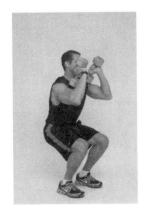

If you are not able to perform the required number of reps with the
weights, use your body weight only and do all 15 reps.

STIFF-LEG DEAD LIFTS

1 set of 15 reps with 10-pound dumbbells

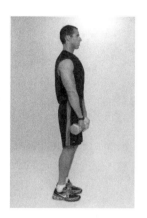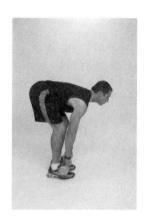

LUNGES

1 set of 15 reps with 10-pound dumbbells

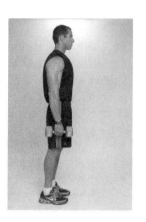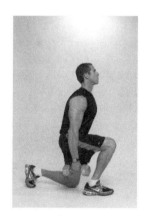

If you are not able to perform the required number of reps with the weights, use your body weight only and do all 15 reps.

PUSH-UPS

1 set of 15 reps on knees

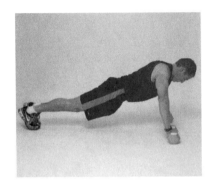 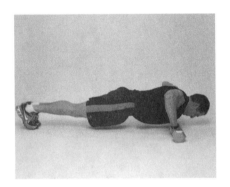

BENT-OVER ROWS

1 set of 15 reps with 12-pound dumbbells

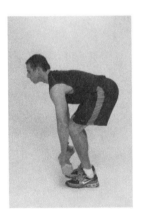 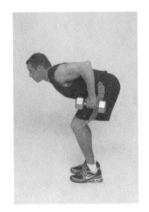

SHOULDER PRESS ON STABILITY BALL

1 set of 15 reps with 10-pound dumbbells

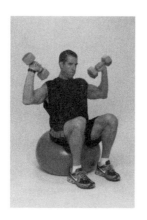 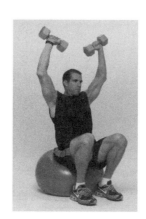

BICEPS CURLS ON STABILITY BALL

1 set of 15 reps with 15-pound dumbbells

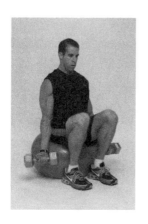 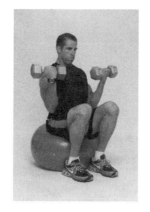

DIPS

1 set of 15 reps with body weight

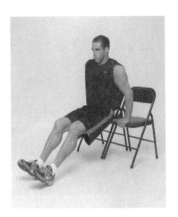 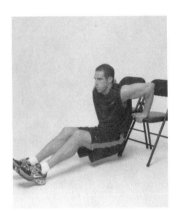

CRUNCHES ON STABILITY BALL

1 set of 20 reps

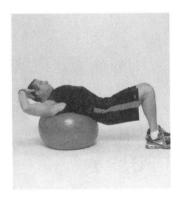 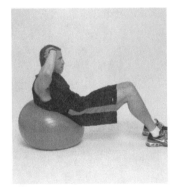

Day 1 Second Set

After completing the entire sequence, rest for one minute. Then go back to the beginning of Day 1's exercises and do:

DUMBBELL SQUATS

1 set of 12 reps with 15-pound dumbbells

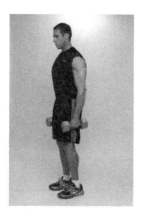 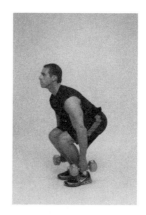

STIFF-LEG DEAD LIFTS

1 set of 12 reps with 15-pound dumbbells

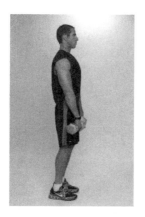 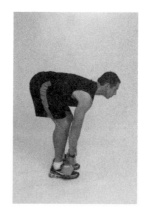

LUNGES

1 set of 12 reps with 15-pound dumbbells

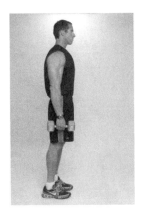 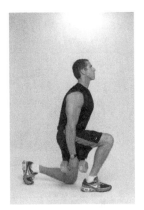

PUSH-UPS

1 set of 12 reps on toes (regular-style push-ups)

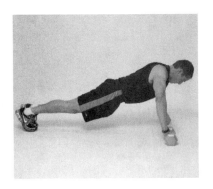 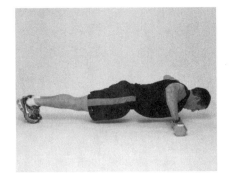

INCLINE PRESS ON STABILITY BALL

1 set of 12 reps with 15-pound dumbbells

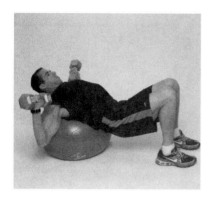 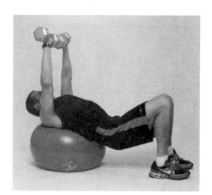

BENT-OVER ROWS

1 set of 12 reps with 20-pound dumbbells

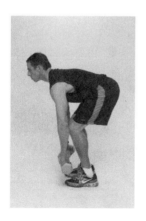 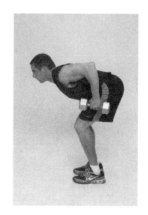

SIDE LATERAL RAISES

1 set of 12 reps with 15-pound dumbbells

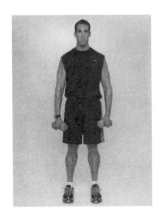 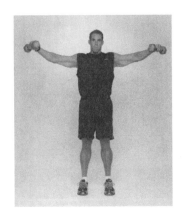

DUMBBELL TRICEPS EXTENSIONS

1 set of 12 reps with 15-pound dumbbells

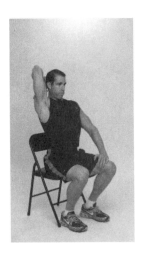 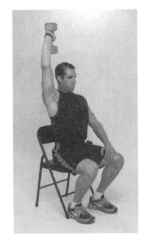

BICEPS CURLS ON STABILITY BALL

1 set of 12 reps with 20-pound dumbbells

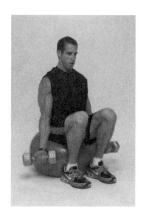 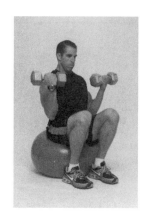

DIPS

1 set of 15 reps with body weight

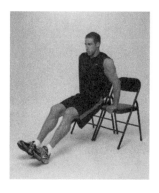 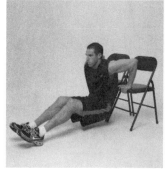

CRUNCHES ON STABILITY BALL

1 set of 20 reps

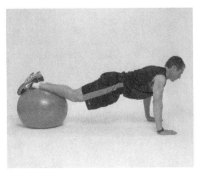 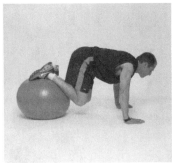

Day 1 Third Set

After completing the entire sequence, rest one minute. Then go back to the beginning for the final set and do:

DUMBBELL SQUATS

1 set of 10 reps with 20-pound dumbbells

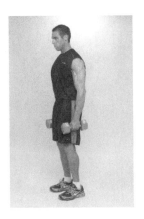 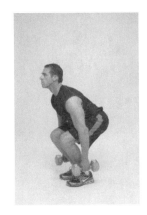

STIFF-LEG DEAD LIFTS

1 set of 10 reps with 20-pound dumbbells

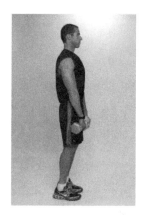 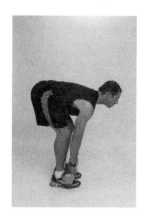

LUNGES

1 set of 10 reps with 20-pound dumbbells

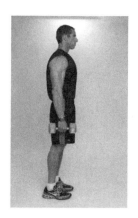 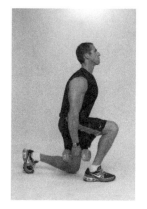

PUSH-UPS

1 set of 12 reps on toes (regular-style push-ups)

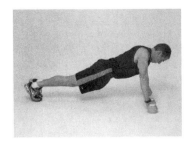
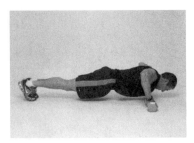

BENT-OVER ROWS

1 set of 12 reps with 20-pound dumbbells

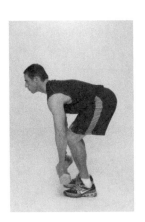
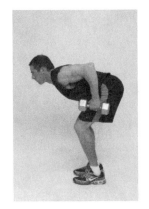

SIDE LATERAL RAISES

1 set of 15 reps with 10-pound dumbbells

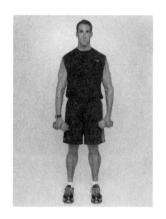 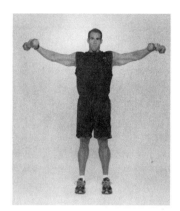

DUMBBELL TRICEPS EXTENSIONS

1 set of 15 reps with 10-pound dumbbells

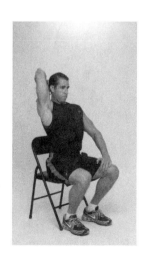 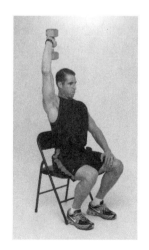

DIPS

1 set of 15 reps with body weight

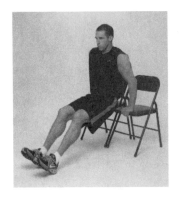 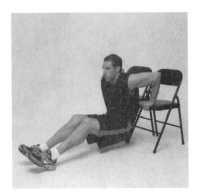

CRUNCHES ON STABILITY BALL

1 set of 10 reps

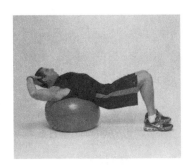 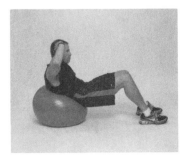

Workout Circuit Day 2

DUMBBELL SQUATS

1 set of 15 reps with 10-pound dumbbells

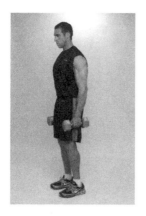 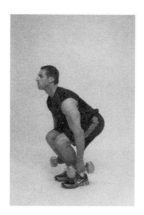

STIFF-LEG DEAD LIFTS

1 set of 15 reps with 10-pound dumbbells

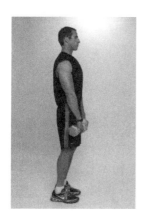 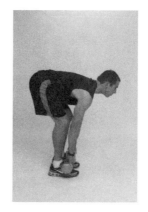

INCLINE PRESS ON STABILITY BALL

1 set of 15 reps with 15-pound dumbbells

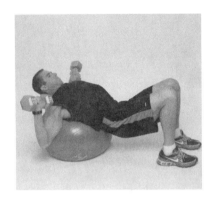 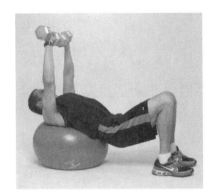

BENT-OVER ROWS

1 set of 15 reps with 15-pound dumbbells

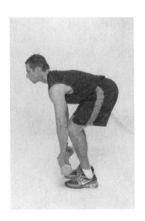 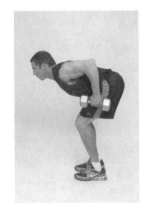

SIDE LATERAL RAISES

1 set of 15 reps with 10-pound dumbbells

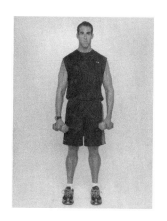 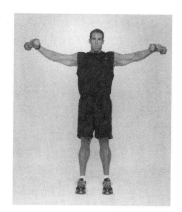

SEATED DUMBBELL TRICEPS EXTENSIONS

1 set of 15 reps with 10-pound dumbbells

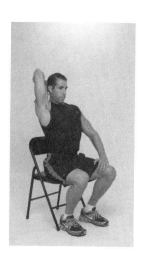 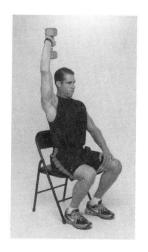

BICEPS CURLS ON STABILITY BALL

1 set of 15 reps with 15-pound dumbbells

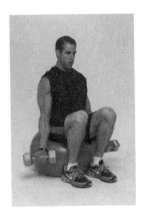 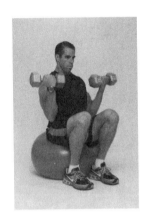

DIPS

1 set of 15 reps with body weight

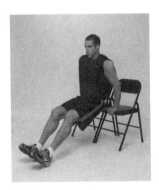 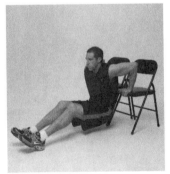

REVERSE CRUNCHES ON STABILITY BALL

1 set of 10 reps

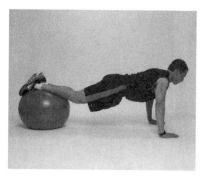 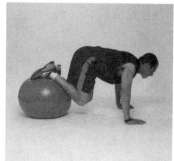

Day 2 Second Set

After completing the entire sequence, rest one minute. Then go back to the beginning of Day 2's exercises and do:

DUMBBELL SQUATS

12 reps with 15-pound dumbbells

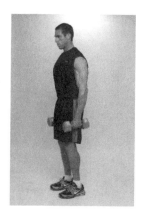 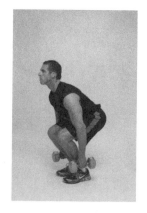

STIFF-LEG DEAD LIFTS

12 reps with 1 pound dumbbells

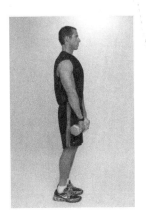 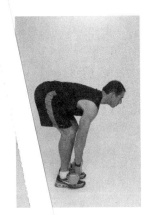

INCLINE PRESS ON STABILITY BALL

12 reps with 20-pound dumbbells

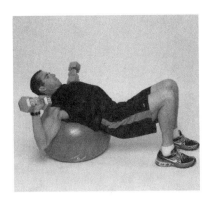 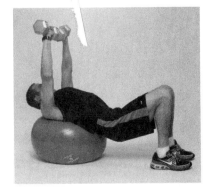

BENT-OVER ROWS

12 reps with 20-pound dumbbells

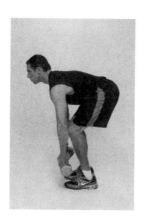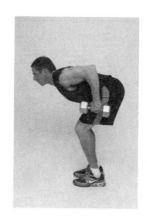

SIDE LATERAL RAISES

12 reps with 15-pound dumbbells

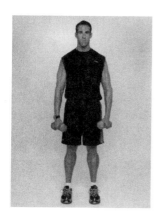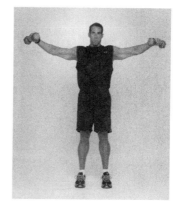

SEATED DUMBBELL TRICEPS EXTENSIONS

12 reps with 15-pound dumbbells

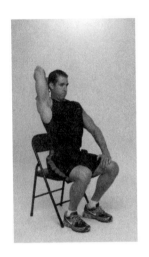 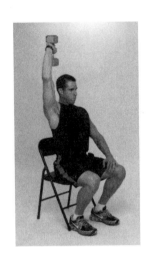

BICEPS CURLS ON STABILITY BALL

12 reps with 20-pound dumbbells

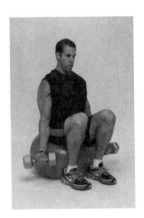 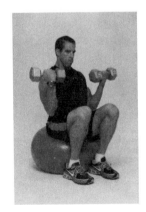

DIPS

12 reps with body weight

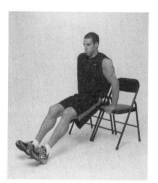 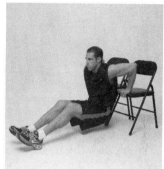

Day 2 Third Set

After completing the entire sequence, rest for one minute. Then go back to the beginning for the final set and do:

DUMBBELL SQUATS

10 reps with 20-pound dumbbells

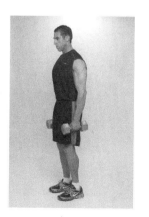 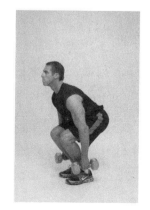

STIFF-LEG DEAD LIFTS

10 reps with 20-pound dumbbells

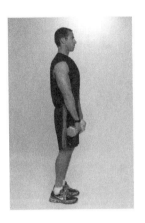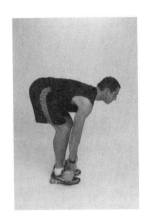

INCLINE PRESS ON STABILITY BALL

12 reps with 20-pound dumbbells

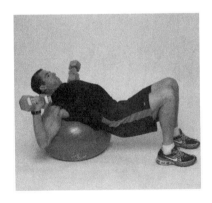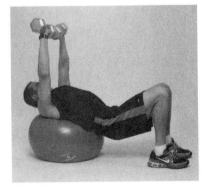

BENT-OVER ROWS

12 reps with 20-pound dumbbells

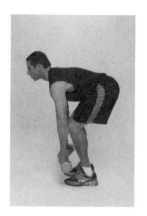 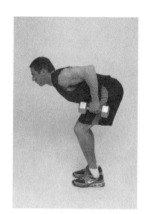

SIDE LATERAL RAISES

12 reps with 15-pound dumbbells

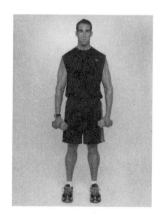 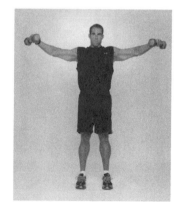

SEATED DUMBBELL TRICEPS EXTENSIONS

10 reps with 20-pound dumbbells

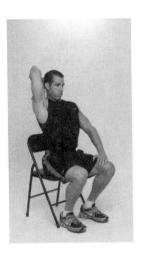 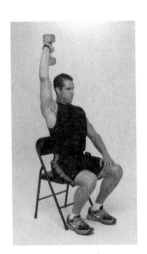

Workout Circuit Day 3

WALL SQUATS USING STABILITY BALL

1 set of 20 reps with body weight

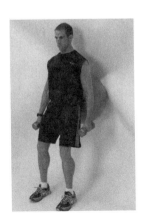 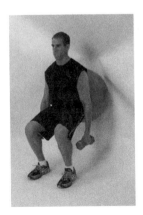

LUNGES

1 set of 15 reps with body weight

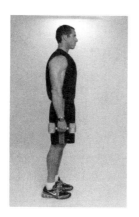 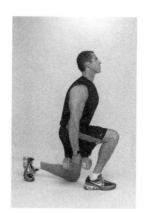

PUSH-UPS

1 set of 15 reps on knees

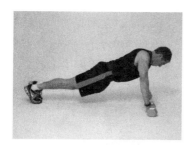 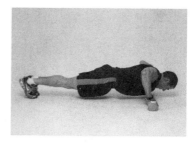

INCLINE PRESS ON STABILITY BALL

1 set of 15 reps with 15-pound dumbbells

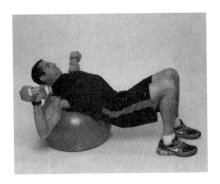 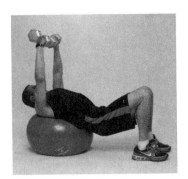

BENT-OVER ROWS

1 set of 15 reps with 15-pound dumbbells

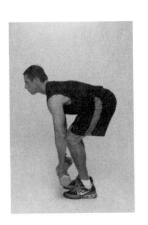 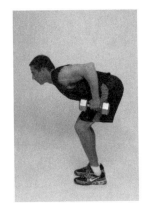

SHOULDER PRESS ON STABILITY BALL

1 set of 15 reps with 10-pound dumbbells

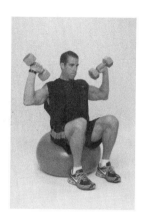 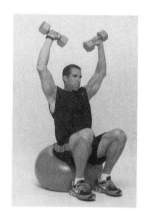

BICEPS CURLS ON STABILITY BALL

1 set of 15 reps with 15-pound dumbbells

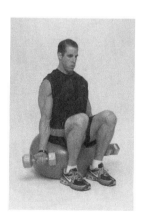 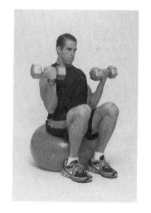

DIPS

1 set of 15 reps with body weight

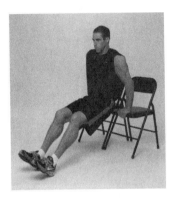 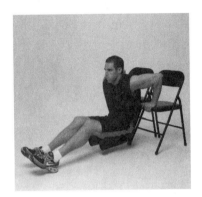

CRUNCHES ON STABILITY BALL

1 set of 20 reps

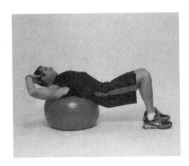 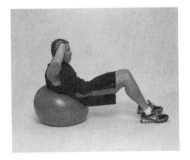

Day 3 Second Set

After completing the entire sequence, rest one minute. Then go back to the beginning of Day 3's exercises and do:

WALL SQUATS USING STABILITY BALL

20 reps with body weight only

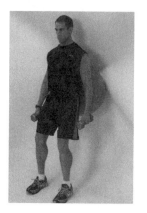 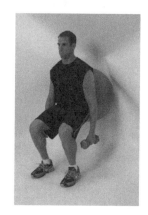

LUNGES

15 reps with body weight only

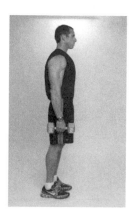 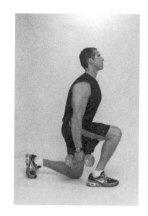

PUSH-UPS

12 reps on toes (regular-style push-ups)

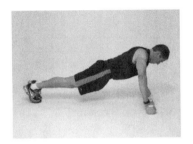
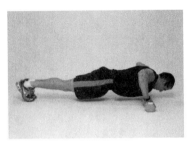

INCLINE PRESS ON STABILITY BALL

12 reps with 20-pound dumbbells

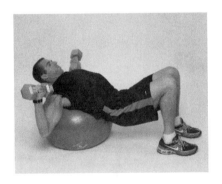
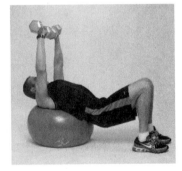

BENT-OVER ROWS

12 reps with 20-pound dumbbells

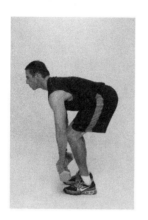 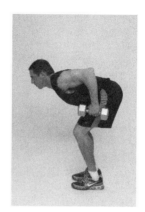

SHOULDER PRESS ON STABILITY BALL

12 reps with 15-pound dumbbells

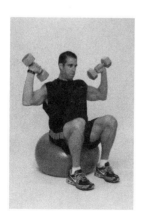 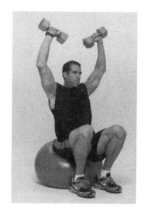

BICEPS CURLS ON STABILITY BALL

12 reps with 20-pound dumbbells

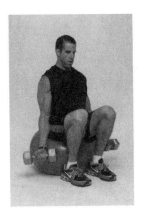 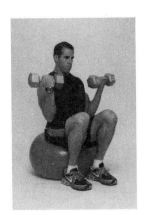

DIPS

12 reps with body weight

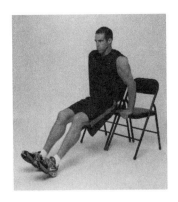 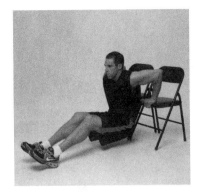

CRUNCHES ON STABILITY BALL

20 reps

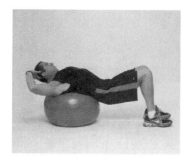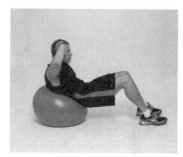

Day 3 Third Set

After completing the entire sequence, rest one minute. Then go back to the beginning for the final set and do:

WALL SQUATS USING STABILITY BALL

20 reps with body weight only

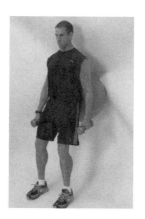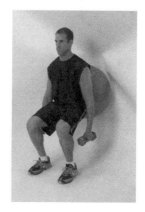

PUSH-UPS

12 reps on toes (regular-style push-ups)

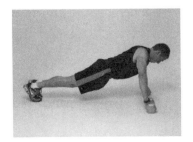 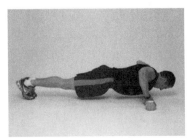

INCLINE PRESS ON STABILITY BALL

12 reps with 20-pound dumbbells

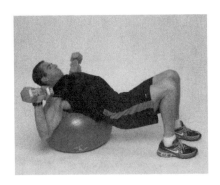 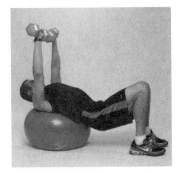

BENT-OVER ROWS

12 reps with 20-pound dumbbells

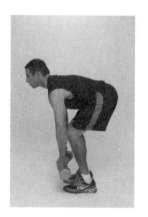 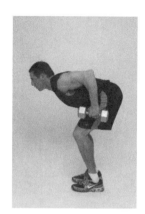

SHOULDER PRESS ON STABILITY BALL

12 reps with 15-pound dumbbells

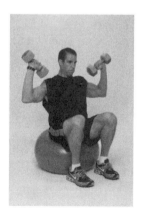 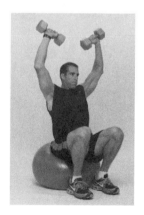

CHAPTER 10

KEEPING YOUR NEW BUFF BODY

We must use time as a tool, not as a crutch.

John F. Kennedy

You've worked hard, you've followed the plan, and you're seeing results. The hard part is over, right? Wrong! Unfortunately, after achieving their goals, many people go back to their old habits and end up in a cycle of dieting/overeating/dieting. The sad news is that many of them end up gaining more weight than they lost while on their diet or weight-loss program.

The secret to keeping it off and maintaining your buff body is to stay on the program. I know it can be challenging and, yes, everybody "cheats" sometimes, but some little tips can help you stay on track and motivated for the long haul.

1   Avoid procrastination by having your workout bag or weights ready to go.

2   Remind yourself how far you've come by keeping a "before" picture handy or your "before" weight posted.

3   Document your success in a fitness log that includes your weight, how much cardio you completed, and how much you lifted.

4   Remind yourself that success is not only shown on the scale, but also in how you feel.

5   Focus on the end result. Imagine what you'll be doing and how you'll look if you stay on the plan.

The Fat Police: Resisting Temptation

The easiest way to stay on track is to stay on the program. But face it, we're all going to fall off the fitness wagon once in a while. The trick is to not lag too far behind by making smart choices even when you're being a "bad" dad rather than a buff dad.

I've been on the *Buff Dad* program for three years now, so believe me when I tell you that I've done it all. Yes, I'm guilty of taking three free days in a row and enjoying pigging out on everything under the sun. Of course, I paid for it later when I put on 8 pounds and had to work my buff dad butt off trying to lose them again. Believe me, just because you're buff one day, it doesn't mean you're immune to putting the weight back on if you go all out. Your metabolism might be better than it was when you were a fat dad, but it can't burn bags of potato chips, burgers, and fries like they were nothing.

I've also skipped the gym every once in a while because I was too tired or too lazy. Then there were times that I just didn't care and did whatever I wanted. Those were the hardest times because not only was I already in a bad place, but by not taking care of myself, I plunged further into my hole of self-pity while getting fatter by the hour.

Being human, I'd love to blame my job, my son, and even my wife for my weaknesses, but I've finally come to the sad conclusion that when I sway from the path of the buff, it is nobody's fault but my own. Surprisingly, when I told my wife this life-changing revelation, she just rolled her eyes. Apparently, she knew this all along, and I was the only one who couldn't see the truth—or as I like to say, I couldn't see the calories for the chips.

While I look buff today, I'm far from perfect, and it wasn't easy getting where I am. Even now I have days when I'm tempted to give in and order a large milkshake with a side order of fries. Basically, no matter how much you work out, you're always going to be the average guy who has to struggle with his weight every day of his life in order to maintain a certain level of fitness. The faster you realize this, the easier staying on the program will become. Psychologically, you'll realize that being tempted doesn't mean you're a failure or that you can't do it; all it means is that you are human and everyone has the same temptations in life. Think about it: if nobody was tempted to eat a Big Mac or supersized fries, the fast-food industry wouldn't be as popular as it is. Whether you admit it or not, you are a part of American pop culture, born and bred on fast food, advertising, and convenience.

The other thing you have to accept is that men tend to talk big, but deep down we're always ready to take the easy way out. What I had to learn is that giving in to eating fattening foods and sugary treats every day isn't the easy way; it's actually the hard way. Every time you cave in to your cravings, it pushes you backward; in the end you have to work harder to get where you want to be.

What all of us fat dads need is our own personal fat security guard. Life would be so much easier if I had a guy armed with a big stick watching everything I put into my mouth and ready to whack me whenever I reached for a slab of chocolate cake or fried chicken.

Unfortunately, unless your spouse and coworkers are secret sadists, no one will grab the big stick and monitor what you consume except yourself. You have to be your own fat police. You're responsible for your own fat, including the love handles that hang over your belt. The good news is that the following wisdom will help you stay on track and stay buff.

Be a Master Planner

Plan your meals, and I mean *every single meal,* including the snacks. It's much less tempting to cheat if you have your breakfast, lunch, and dinner planned. Planning also means shopping with a grocery list. Having healthy food in the house ready for dinner means you'll be less tempted to pick up something on the way home or to order in. For example, instead of grabbing a doughnut or bagel at the office, check out Eggology On the Go (www.eggology.com). Eggology on the Go is four egg whites in a microwave-safe container. Zap it in the microwave, and you have a delicious hot and healthy breakfast. Just add some fruit and you have a complete *Buff Dad* breakfast.

Realize Your Imperfections

Acknowledge when you fail, and then go right back on the program. We're all going to cheat sometimes. Tell yourself it's okay, and then start the program again. Don't wait until Monday or the next morning. Begin right after you've finished "being bad." While cheating is never a good thing, getting back on track will help reduce some of the negative repercussions.

Avoid the Binge Fest

Okay, so you caved and ate a bag of chips. Get over it and move on. Don't tell yourself you've ruined the diet and you'll start again tomorrow. Continuing to eat everything in sight for the rest of the day will only lead to serial bingeing, and you could end up putting on much more weight.

Always Have Your Weekly Free Meal

The free meal not only gives you something to look forward to, but will help reduce the cravings. Plus, if you do have a craving, you can count down the days until you can finally eat what you want.

Trick Your Taste Buds

If you do have a craving and absolutely can't resist, look for a low-fat option. This doesn't mean eating a pile of lettuce when you really want a burger. The secret is to fight temptation by tricking your taste buds and making your mind and body believe they got what they wanted.

So if you're craving a burger, think about what you're craving. Is it the texture, the taste, or the way it feels in your stomach? Then, instead of caving in to the temptation and running to a fast-food restaurant, make something similar that will satisfy the craving, such as a turkey burger if it's the texture you want, or a low-fat tuna melt if it's the melted cheese that's going to satisfy you.

CRAVING CRUSHER

Instead of potato chips, try munching on a half cup of green olives. Olives satisfy salt cravings, plus they are filled with omega-3 oils that help your body recover more quickly from exercise by reducing inflammation.

Maintaining Your Goals

After four weeks of working out and eating right, you'll be well on your way to becoming the buff dad you've always dreamed of being. But what happens when you reach your goal? What do you do when you're "buff enough"?

The answer is maintenance, which doesn't mean you get to slack off. In order to maintain your muscle tone and keep up your lean look, you'll still need to lift weights and do cardio. In fact, the best thing to do is go back to week one and start the program again, this time adding more weight so that you don't plateau. Each time you go through the program, you'll be stronger, leaner, and buffer. You'll be more likely to maintain your success if you have a plan like the *Buff Dad* program rather than winging it on your own.

While you don't get a vacation from the workout portion of the program, where you do get a break is in the food area. Up until the time that you've reached your goal, you've been slowly losing fat and gaining muscle. Even those of you who might have experienced a slight weight gain when you first started putting on muscle eventually discovered that you've lost both fat and inches off your body by sticking to the program. So now that you've reached your goal, you'll want to stop losing and start maintaining. To do this, you'll have to increase your calories.

Don't get too excited. Increasing your calories doesn't mean you get to eat cake, fries, and fat-drenched burgers every day. In order to maintain what you have and keep your body working like a well-oiled machine, you'll need to keep eating the approved *Buff Dad* testosterone-enhancing foods on the list. You just get to eat a little more of them.

So how much more can you eat? While I would love to give you a set amount of food, the answer lies with you. Most guys will be able to eat up to 500 extra calories a day and not gain weight, but depending on your genetic makeup and metabolism, you may only be able to get away with an extra 200 calories. After a couple of days of trial and error, you'll figure out what you can get away with and what you can't. Just be careful and make sure the numbers on the scale don't slowly creep up on you.

Top-Ten Diet Mistakes

1. Not eating enough calories.

2. Too much cardio.

3. Working out too hard.

4. Working only your "favorite" muscles.

5. Skipping the post-workout stretch.

6. Not eating every three hours.

7. Doing the exact same workout every day.

8. Not eating enough testosterone-rich foods.

9. Working out only a couple of times a week.

10. Not getting enough sleep.

Dealing with Emotional Eating

W e all got fat for a reason. While eating too much and doing too little were the physical reasons we gained the weight, whether we realize it or not, many of us fat dads were eating for other reasons. Studies show that some of the more common reasons we eat are that we're bored or upset, which leads to binge eating, which leads to becoming more upset and frustrated, which leads to more eating.

While the *Buff Dad* program can help you lose weight and become lean, working out like a demon doesn't deal with the hidden reasons for why you got fat in the first place. To understand why you gained weight, you first have to figure out why you eat. In fact, because emotional eating is so common, you probably fall into one of the three following categories.

The Habit-Eater

Do you find yourself coming home from work and going straight to the fridge—even though you're not hungry or you just ate? Do you find that when you watch a movie, you must have something to munch on? Do you find you need a little something sweet at the end of the meal to finish it off? Do you always purchase a "treat" with your coffee when you go to the cafeteria or to Starbucks? If you answered yes to any of these questions, you might be a habit-eater.

Just like a smoker addicted to nicotine, eating becomes a bad habit for many people, but instead of getting cancer, your habit is making you fat, which can lead to heart disease, cholesterol problems, and other serious health concerns.

The solution is to break up the routine, simply exchanging one action for another—preferably a healthier one. For example, when you come home from work, instead of going to the fridge, get in the habit of pouring yourself a glass of water instead.

The Emotional Binger

Just because you don't cry during Hallmark commercials doesn't mean you're not an emotional binger. People associate food with a lot of things and use it to help them deal with stress, sadness, loneliness, anger, and frustration. Even happiness and excitement can cause people to eat. Food can be a source of comfort for the trying times, but it also can be used as a reward for the good times.

The first thing to remember is that if you are an emotional eater, you're not alone. For many of us, food is part of our society. We're brought up associating food with good times, family love, and other positive moments in our lives. If you think about it, every celebration has some sort of food associated with it: birthday and wedding cakes, Thanksgiving dinners, Fourth of July BBQs, and holiday parties. Of course, the food associated with all those good times isn't low in fat.

While the occasional celebration with food is okay, having a little food treat a few times a week to help you cope could keep you spiraling mentally and physically for the rest of your life. Not only does binge eating make you fat, but because the foods most often binged on are usually high in sugar or fat, you wreak havoc on the body's glycerin levels so you're in a constant state of emotional mountain highs and valley lows. While you're boosting yourself with a decadent chocolate sundae and feeling wonderful, once the sugar is processed, your body plunges to lower-than-normal glycerin levels, making you feel run-down and tired. Of course, this is the last way you want to feel if you're already stressed or depressed, so you end up bingeing again to re-elevate your energy.

To conquer this problem, make a plan in advance with some alternative solutions to deal with stress or whatever emotion triggers your binges. You may want to treat yourself to a massage or go out to the driving range and whack a bucket of balls. Remember, these feelings will pass. You just have to keep yourself busy during the tempting stages.

The Boredom Muncher

This little devil describes me. I'll munch at work if I'm having a slow day or working on a project I don't find particularly interesting. I'll munch in the mall at the food court while waiting for my wife to finish her shopping. I'll even munch while my son is playing soccer and I'm cheering him on along the sidelines. Basically, I'll eat anytime and anywhere.

The way to deal with this problem is to never be bored. I know, that's asking too much, so I've come up with a better solution: don't keep foods around that tempt you.

If you stop to think about it, when you're bored you don't sit down and eat a head of lettuce with a side of tomatoes. If you're like me, you combat your boredom with potato chips, pizza, soft drinks, and other fast and convenient foods that taste good going down, but look bad on the scale.

My wife has already learned not to buy anything that comes in a bag, such as cookies, chips, or nuts, as I'm the type of person who likes to finish the whole thing off in one sitting. It doesn't matter if it's the bonus bag with 25 percent more chips and is meant to feed a party of thirty. I can't stop until it's completely gone.

Unfortunately, not buying snack foods isn't enough to dissuade me when the time hits. That's because I'm not only the Boredom Muncher, but I'm creative with my food choices.

I remember one time I was so desperate for junk food that I must have looked in the refrigerator at least thirty times trying to find something to eat. Unfortunately, all that was in there was healthy food. And while I silently cursed my spouse for listening to me and not buying anything with fat in it, I wasn't about to defrost and broil a chicken breast to fill my needs.

Even with nothing in the house, I wasn't about to give up. In my desperation, I ended up improvising by spreading peanut butter on a celery stalk and then dipping it in my son's chocolate syrup.

I realized I had a problem. I had taken my boredom bingeing a step too far.

To get control, I now have a picture of the fat me posted on our refrigerator. It's a constant reminder of who I was and who I could be again if I don't stay in control. Oh . . . and my wife is also no longer allowed to buy chocolate syrup.

Overcoming Fitness Plateaus

If you've been doing the program diligently, you've probably been seeing results. But what happens if the results stop showing and you get stuck in a holding pattern?

Don't worry. Fitness and weight plateaus can happen to anyone. It doesn't mean your body has stopped progressing and is as good as it's going to get. Instead, it means that your body is ready for the next challenge.

There are three surefire ways to beat fitness plateaus and boost yourself into the next level. The good news is you probably only need to do one out of the three options in order to get your body back on track.

Double-Check Your Diet

Are you following everything perfectly? If so, try reducing either your free meal to one special treat instead of an all-out calorie extravaganza or cut back on one of your three snacks a day. Keep in mind that even vegetables have calories if you eat too many of them, so make sure your portions are in control.

Increase Your Cardio

You probably hate doing cardio, but it's one of the best things you can do to burn fat quickly. If cutting down on your calories is out of the question, add more cardio to your week by either doing 30 minutes every day (instead of every second day) or increasing your cardio to 45 minutes.

Increase Your Weights

Having more muscle tone also helps you burn more fat. If you're not feeling the burn at the end of the twelfth repetition during your weight-lifting sessions, it's time to increase your resistance by using heavier weights.

The *Buff Dad* Website

The *Buff Dad* website **www.buffdads.com** is a tool for you and other dads on the program who need to stay motivated. I find that one way to truly enjoy your success is to share it with someone else. Don't get me wrong: I'm sure your spouse loves hearing about you talk about yourself all day long, but if you need a little change or decide to give her a break, the website is the perfect place for you to share in cyberspace.

On the site you can share your challenges and success secrets with other buff dads. You can discuss and learn about fitness and diet tips, as well as share advice on fatherhood.

CHAPTER 11

BUFF DAD GUIDE TO FAST-FOOD DINING

It's not whether you get knocked down; it's whether
you get up.

Vince Lombardi

C anada and the United States are known as fast-food nations.
Statistics show that every day, one out of every four people
eats fast food. Unfortunately, if you're one of these people,
you're not only going to be a fat dad forever, but all this eating out is
probably wreaking havoc on your arteries, cholesterol level, and heart.

But avoiding fast food forever isn't the answer either. We all know
eventually you're going to end up at the infamous Golden Arches with
your child, on a family vacation somewhere, or at some sort of party
where the food is in abundance and so are the calories.

So rather than barricading yourself in the comfort of your home and becoming a hermit, I'm going to guide you through the grease-laden world of fast food and help you pick out healthier choices that won't jack up the number on the scale.

Restaurants Are Your Friends

E ven though burgers, fries, pizzas, and other convenience foods most likely were the main reasons you packed on the pounds over the years, the good news is that fast-food havens don't have to be your doom. In fact, over the last few years, the food-service industry has been forced to reconsider what they have on their menus and add healthier options, because we have become more aware of how food drenched in fat, sugar, and calories affects our bodies and have started demanding alternatives.

I'm not saying I was one of these people who really wanted grilled chicken and salad added to the burger menu, but enough of the general public realized that we had become fat enough and voiced their opinion. This new health trend makes it much easier for us guys who want to transform our couch-potato bodies into buff dads.

Because of those health-conscious people before us, healthy choices already exist on many menus. Plus, because they are becoming more popular, the selections have evolved from boring salads to stuff you'd actually want to eat. You just have to look past your normal meal combos to see them.

Some ways to order healthy include:

→ Order the single-patty burger instead of the triple-patty.

→ Order grilled chicken sandwiches instead of burgers.

→ Ask for whole-wheat rolls.

→ Ask for a slice of fruit on the side instead of coleslaw.

→ Order salads with the dressing on the side.

→ Choose balsamic vinegar as your salad dressing.

→ Order wraps instead of hot beef or club sandwiches.

→ Order water instead of soft drinks.

→ Never, ever supersize!

→ Skip gravy and cheese whenever possible.

→ Avoid breaded chicken, fish, French fries, and onion rings.

Conquering Office Lunch Temptations

For those of you who aren't going to the gym during lunch and working off the pounds, you may have to deal with the problem of office lunches.

Brown bagging isn't always convenient, especially if your office environment is one where everyone orders in or eats in a cafeteria. Rather than being a water-cooler outcast, you can choose smart alternatives and still lose weight.

Sandwiches are the easiest lunch menu item to make low-fat and high in protein. Your best bet is to choose turkey breast and specify the number of slices you want. Although it will be tempting to let them dump that giant pile of meat on the bun, you'll probably want to limit it to two slices of meat. Another way to cut fat and calories is to opt for mustard over mayonnaise and ask for whole-wheat bread.

There are also low-fat choices when it comes to popular lunchtime ethnic foods. Chinese chicken with broccoli is a good alternative compared to black bean sauce or breaded meats. In Italian restaurants, select pastas with marinara sauces or tossed in olive oil. Again, stay away from fried or breaded entrées such as veal or chicken parmigiana, and skip the cheese whenever possible.

Eight Satisfying Fast-Food Choices (less than 10g of fat)

1. McDonald's Chicken McGrill with no mayo (4.5g of fat)

2. Subway 6" Roast Beef on whole-wheat bread and no sauce (5g of fat)

3. Wendy's Ultimate Chicken Grill Sandwich (7g of fat)

4. McDonald's Hamburger (9g of fat)

5. Wendy's Jr. Hamburger (9g of fat)

6. KFC Original Recipe Chicken Breast with breading and skin removed (4.5g of fat)

7. Pizza Hut Fit 'N Delicious Chicken & Veggie Pizza (2 slices for 9g of fat)

8. Taco Bell Fresco Grilled Steak Soft Tacos (2 for 10g of fat)

The *Buff Dad* Fat Builders

Condiments and side orders are the worst offenders on the menu when it comes to being healthy. In addition to butter and mayonnaise, cheese sauce, tartar sauce, and gravy are some of the most unhealthy items you can consume, but they can be replaced easily with low-fat alternatives.

For example, instead of smothering butter on your rolls, ask for olive oil and balsamic vinegar. Another healthy suggestion is to skip the cheese on burgers and sandwiches. Chances are you don't taste it anyway so why add the calories?

Buff Dad Smart Alternatives

Broth-based soups	Veggie or turkey burger
Whole-grain breads	Baked potato
Fruit as a side or garnish	Tossed salad
Peel-and-eat shrimp	Baked beans
Blackened chicken sandwich	Sherbet

Making Your Own Fast Food

Chicken nuggets, fried chicken, French fries, and onion rings are some of the most popular convenience foods and the ones we tend to crave. The bad news is that these items are also the most fattening. But there is hope. An easy way to transform a potentially unhealthy food into a healthier variety is to bake it rather than throwing it in the deep fryer.

Egg rolls, tortillas, chicken nuggets, and French fries are examples of foods that taste just as good oven-baked as they do fried. Baking also provides you with the opportunity to get a little creative in the kitchen. Instead of using traditional potatoes, use sweet potatoes (or yams) or brush regular potatoes with olive oil and sprinkle with spices such as a Cajun blend to add a little spice. Also, when baking, you can leave the skin on for extra color and fiber.

Other healthier cooking techniques include making thin-crust pizzas with low-fat cheese. However, if you're going to buy a frozen pizza, the American Dietetic Association recommends choosing one with 350 to 450 calories per serving and around 10 grams of total fat. Beef up the slices by adding extra frozen green peppers, mushrooms, or even broccoli before popping the pie into the oven. Chopping up a few cloves of testosterone-building garlic and adding it to the finished pizza adds extra zing, but only do this if your spouse is having pizza, too. Nothing is worse than one-sided garlic breath—no matter how much testosterone you have coursing through your nearly muscled body.

Remember . . . no matter what you make at home, don't forget to watch your serving size. Sometimes it is a lot smaller than you think.

BUFF DAD TIP

Ask for extra sauce on your pizza or even some on the side to dip your crust in. It's low in fat, and tomatoes are known for their ability to reduce the risk of prostate cancer.

CHAPTER 12

ENJOYING FATHERHOOD AS A *BUFF DAD*

Well done is better than well said.

Benjamin Franklin

You've done it. You're a buff dad. Now what? Now that you're fit, it's time to bring your new lifestyle and good health to your entire family by doing activities with them. Does that mean you have to drag your son or daughter with you to the gym every day? Not at all. While taking them to the gym may keep them in shape, your coolness factor as a dad might go down a couple of notches. Instead, you can do a number of other activities that are much more fun and will bring your family closer together.

Enjoying the Great Outdoors

The outdoors is a great way to stay in shape while creating a healthy lifestyle for your family. Going on a bike ride, whether it's through your own neighborhood or on a cycling path, is an excellent way to spend quality time with your kids—plus it's inexpensive and something most kids love to do. But don't limit the experience to just going around the block a couple of times. Really get into it by transforming your family vacations, weekends, and other events into bike-friendly adventures. Nearby campgrounds, parks, and trails often have paths created that are perfect for family biking.

Another way to get your family excited about biking is having them help plan the trip. Depending on their age, your kids can take turns researching bike trails on the Internet or planning picnic meals and snacks for the ride.

I just have one word of advice when planning a cycling trip: remember to keep your family's fitness level in mind. You may have been working out every day for the last month or so and are ready to bike for hours, but your child is much smaller. They have smaller legs and a smaller heart, and they get tired more quickly.

In other words, don't plan a forty-mile bike ride. Not only will this not be fun for your child, but they probably won't want to go biking again with you. You want to make fitness something they enjoy doing and not something they consider punishment or torture.

If biking is not for you, don't sweat it. You can do many other activities as a family. One that everyone can do is walking.

Never underestimate the power of your own two feet and adventures you can take your kids on. Where you go is up to you. You might want to start in your own neighborhood on a daily after-school or after-dinner walk. Once that gets boring for the kids, you can branch into other areas of the city.

Just like biking, you can turn walking into an exciting excursion by planning weekend getaways that involve hiking or seeing historical places. Of course, not every kid is going to find walking exciting. If your child's attention span isn't that long, try making the walking trips part of a game. Give them an "I spy" list and have them shoot pictures or make it a scavenger hunt and have them look for clues during the walk. Award prizes for the person who finds the most clues.

One final idea is to check into local attractions and events. Many city zoos have special walking events in the off-season. Others set up cross-country skiing trails in the winter months that go through the open areas of the zoo. While most of the tropical animals are moved inside, some of the outdoor animals such as buffalo are still out, making the skiing extra fun.

Another family-fitness idea is to join charity events. The American Heart Association has yearly Heart Walks that are perfect for families. You can also search the Internet for family-friendly hiking trails near you.

Buff Dad Meets Sporty Dad

Become the dad everyone wishes was their own by either playing sports with your kids or coaching a youth team. Basketball, volleyball, soccer, and football are team sports that turn getting fit into a buddy activity. Even if you can't play with your kids, you can be there to help practice by playing family versions of their sport in the backyard.

Many times as your kids get older, it's hard to stay connected with them. One way to fix this is to find an activity that you both like and join it together. This could be golf, karate, bird-watching, Rollerblading, or even motocross racing.

But if your child isn't into organized sports, look for other activities you can do together, such as fishing trips from a canoe rather than a motorboat. Really, when it comes down to it, it doesn't matter how old your child is. Somewhere out there, there is a fun fitness activity waiting for you and your family to do together. Plus, the bond you create now will be something your child will remember for the rest of his or her life.

Five Simple Ways to Become a Buff Family

1. Replace 30 minutes of TV time each day with physical activity.

2. Consider walking to the store, playground, or school instead of driving whenever possible.

3. Buy toys that promote physical activity such as balls, jump ropes, and bicycles.

4. Designate areas indoors and outdoors where rolling, jumping, climbing, and tumbling are allowed.

5. Use physical activity, rather than food, as a reward (family goes hiking or family canoe day).

Setting Free the Buff Romantic in You

While being a buff dad means you can be healthier and do more things with your children, there is more to being a dad than hanging out with the kids. Being a good dad also means being a good husband. In other words, when planning quality fitness time with your child, don't forget to include some special moments for your wife.

We all look forward to those special weekends when we can leave the kids with Grandma and be alone with the mother of our children. While I'm sure you can come up with plenty of physical activities you can do to fill this quality time, there are others that will actually get you out of the bedroom—and still keep your spouse happy.

I admit that after I lost all my dad fat, I was completely into my new lifestyle. Unfortunately, my wife was not. Don't get me wrong. She loved the new buff me, but she didn't really want to change her life just because I was into being buff. Don't ask me why, but she didn't think watching me lift weights and sweat was time well spent, and she definitely didn't find it romantic.

So because she wasn't about to hang out with me at the gym, I had to come up with fitness activities that included her and, of course, made her feel special. One of these was a biking wine tour that I found online.

It sounds a little bit strange to mix something that requires balance with drinking, but believe me, my wife loved it. The tour group provided bicycles and over the next four hours led us on a tour of three vineyards. It was about ten miles of leisurely biking in total, which kept me on track with my cardio, but because we stopped and sampled the wines along the way, my wife never complained—not even once. In fact, she thought the whole thing was romantic. So I not only got to work out, but I earned mega-points in the husband category.

Other romantic, yet fitness-enhancing activities include going for walks together, sunset canoe trips, and, of course, dancing.

Stop groaning and put on your dancing shoes. A lot of women love a man who can dance and find it a big turn-on. So if you've got any rhythm in you, this is the time to use it to your advantage and enroll in weekly lessons. It's great cardio, and the hour you spend on the dance floor will help keep your marriage connected as it's something you both do together.

Just One Last Thing . . .

One final word of encouragement before I let you go to start living your new buff life. Remember to take every day one step at a time. Even after being on the plan for a couple of years, I still have days when I fall back to my old ways. I'm no saint, but I have learned the secret of staying buff: forgive yourself and move on.

Remember, in the *Buff Dad* program, you are working on four different aspects of your life:

1 **Your physical fitness.** Let's face it. The reason you've decided to do the program is to lose weight, increase your muscle mass, and look more toned, which is why my proven thirty-minute *Buff Dad* Workout Blitz is the core of the program.

Specifically designed to maximize performance and increase tone, each workout enables you to speed up your metabolism, get firm, and burn fat as efficiently as possible.

2 **Your eating habits.** Working out is not enough. In order to maximize your workout and increase your results, you'll learn how to fuel your body effectively.

The *Buff Dad* Dietary Plan is easy to follow and has simple guidelines. You will never feel deprived, nor will you have the hassle of counting calories, buying special foods, or cutting out entire food groups. Learn how to eat and feel satisfied by eating foods that enhance your testosterone levels.

These testosterone-boosting foods help your muscles work more efficiently during workouts, allowing you to tone your body faster in the least amount of time. Plus, they make you feel full and have the added benefit of increasing your sex drive. It's a win/win situation all around.

3 **Your emotional and mental fitness.** So now that you've got the physical sides of eating and toning down to an art form, it's time to handle the hard part: your emotional and mental health.

As a guy, I hated to admit that I'm vulnerable, and there was no way I was ready to admit that food had an emotional impact on me. But it did.

I didn't get fat overnight. As much as it seemed as if I woke up and suddenly couldn't button up my pants, getting to that point was gradual. It was a process that involved a number of factors, including habit, lifestyle, emotional stress, and other factors that were going on in my life.

Each person is unique, and losing weight is not always easy. There will be times you want to give up, cheat, or even fall back to your old ways.

The good news is you won't go through it alone. I've been there and know exactly what you'll be feeling and some of the obstacles you'll need to overcome.

Much of the weight I gained after my son was born developed out of bad habits. Even though many of them seemed harmless, they were slowing me down. I needed to break them before I really moved forward. Some of them, such as simply going to the fridge as soon as I got home from work, were the reason that I would plateau on the program and get frustrated. The great thing is that once I recognized which habits were holding me back, I was able to finally reach my final goal.

4 **Your family life.** As a buff dad myself, the more time I can spend with my son, the better. The last thing you want to do is spend all your time getting buff and end up reducing the time you spend with your child and your spouse.

The *Buff Dad* Dietary Plan also can be used for family meals. Mealtime is key bonding time for many families, so it doesn't make sense to have one meal for you and a second for the rest of the family. Besides being nutritious and tasty, the meals are perfect for everyone in the entire family.

Twenty-Eight Days to a Buff Dad

Believe me, if I can be a buff dad, you can be one, too. Whenever you think you can't, go back and read over the plan. It's simple, it's easy, and it's doable. Plus, you're going to see results in less than a month. Nothing beats seeing the numbers drop on the scale or seeing your tummy slowly transform from flab to firm. Just count down the days, and if you follow the workout and the dietary plan exactly, you'll lose the weight and see a drastic change in your body. I guarantee it!

Now go out there and become the buff dad you always wanted to be!

CHAPTER 13

BUFF DAD
RECIPES

A life spent making mistakes is not only more honorable,
but more useful than a life spent doing nothing.

George Bernard Shaw

hile you have to watch how much you consume, the great
thing about the *Buff Dad* Dietary Plan is that there is no
calorie counting, no foods that are forbidden, and no special supplements. I know how busy you are, and the last thing you
need is to complicate your life with complicated meals.

This is where my years of experience as a dietitian come in handy.
Over the past decade, I've worked as a nutritionist for the California
Angels baseball team, the Chicago Bears and the Oakland Raiders
football teams, as well as with world-famous athletes such as Charles

Oakley, J. T. Snow, Jim Abbott, Gary DiSarcina, and Sean Rooks of the Los Angeles Clippers. In other words, I know what works and what doesn't work.

I also know what foods you need to eat to feel satisfied while losing weight and gaining muscle. But most important, I know how to make low-fat, testosterone-filled meals that taste good. Believe me, the last thing you want is a hungry and unsatisfied Charles Oakley chasing after you.

So roll up your sleeves and prepare to dig in to some guilt-free meals that are guaranteed to help you lose weight and boost your muscle-building testosterone levels.

The asterisk (*) denotes muscle-building, testosterone-enhancing food.

BREAKFAST
RECIPES

Protein Power Pancakes

SERVES 2

What you will need:

1 cup uncooked whole-grain oats (non-instant)

1½ cups of Eggology or 6 egg whites*

1 cup fat-free cottage cheese*

¼ tsp vanilla extract

¼ tsp ground cinnamon

2 packets sugar substitute

½ cup sugar-free maple syrup

¼ cup mixed berries

Lightly coat a nonstick skillet or griddle with cooking spray and place over medium heat. In a blender, combine oats, egg whites, cottage cheese, vanilla, cinnamon, and sugar substitute. Blend for about a minute until smooth.

Pour batter onto hot skillet and cook pancake until bubbly on top and dry around the edges. It takes about 3 minutes. Flip and cook the other side until golden brown.

Top pancakes with warm maple syrup and mixed berries.

NUTRITIONAL INFORMATION
Calories: 520 • Calories from Fat: 50
Total Fat: 6g • Saturated Fat: 1g • Dietary Fiber: 16g • Protein: 37g

Buff Dad Breakfast Turk-wich

SERVES 1

What you will need:

1 whole egg*

⅔ cup of Eggology or 3 egg whites*

2 tbsp skim milk

⅛ tsp ground black pepper

2 slices whole-wheat bread

1 slice turkey* (substituting lean ham is acceptable)

1 slice reduced-fat cheddar cheese

Lightly coat a small nonstick skillet with butter-flavored cooking spray and place over medium heat.

In a small mixing bowl, whisk together egg, egg whites, skim milk, and black pepper. Pour the egg mixture into skillet and stir until set. Then remove from skillet and set aside.

Using the same skillet, add one slice of bread. Layer with turkey or ham, cooked eggs, and cheese, then cover with remaining bread slice. Cook over medium heat until bottom slice is brown. Flip sandwich over and cook until cheese is melted and bread is golden brown.

NUTRITIONAL INFORMATION
Calories: 360 • Calories from Fat: 110
Total Fat: 12g • Saturated Fat: 5g • Dietary Fiber: 4g • Protein: 35g

Early-Bird Pizza

SERVES 1

What you will need:

1 whole egg*

⅔ cup of Eggology or 3 egg whites*

2 tbsp salsa, divided

½ green bell pepper, diced

1 slice of onion, chopped

1 pita

1 slice reduced-fat cheddar cheese

In a small mixing bowl, lightly beat egg and egg whites. Add 1 tbsp of salsa and blend well.

Lightly coat a nonstick skillet with cooking spray. Sauté diced bell pepper and onion over medium heat until soft, then add the egg mixture and cook with vegetables until set.

Place pita on a plate and spoon the egg mixture on it. Top with cheese and microwave until the cheese melts. Top the pita pizza with remaining salsa.

NUTRITIONAL INFORMATION
Calories: 390 • Calories from Fat: 110
Total Fat: 12g • Saturated Fat: 5g • Dietary Fiber: 7g • Protein: 31g

Strawberry-Banana Power Shake

SERVES 1

What you will need:

    12 oz cold water

    1 scoop (37.5 grams) of any low-sugar protein powder

    1 small ripe banana

    6 frozen strawberries

Pour cold water in blender, then add protein powder and blend on medium speed for 15 seconds. Add banana, blend. Then add frozen strawberries and blend once more. Pour into a glass and serve.

NUTRITIONAL INFORMATION
Calories: 170 • Calories from Fat: 10
Total Fat: 1g • Saturated Fat: 0g • Dietary Fiber: 3g • Protein: 16g

Mexican Egg Burrito

SERVES 1

What you will need:

1 (8-inch) whole-wheat tortilla

1 whole egg*

⅔ cup of Eggology or 3 egg whites*

1 lettuce leaf

2 tbsp fat-free refried beans*

1 tbsp reduced-fat cheddar cheese, shredded

¼ cup salsa, divided

Lightly coat a nonstick skillet with cooking spray and place over medium heat. Place tortilla in the skillet and warm each side. Place warmed tortilla on a small plate.

Whisk the egg and egg whites together and pour into warmed skillet. Cook until set. Meanwhile, place the lettuce leaf on the tortilla and spread refried beans over leaf. Top beans with cooked eggs, shredded cheese, and 2 tbsp of salsa.

Roll up tortilla and top with remaining salsa.

NUTRITIONAL INFORMATION
Calories: 320 • Calories from Fat: 70
Total Fat: 8g • Saturated Fat: 1.5g • Dietary Fiber: 5g • Protein: 26g

Make-Ahead Oatmeal

SERVES 2

What you will need:

½ cup boiling water

½ cup rolled oats (not 1-minute oats)

1 cup nonfat plain yogurt

¼ cup raisins or dried chopped apricots

2 tbsp natural bran

2 tbsp oat bran

2 tbsp ground flaxseed

1 apple with peel, cored and chopped

1 tsp cinnamon

In a medium bowl, pour boiling water over rolled oats. Let stand until water is absorbed (about 25 minutes). Add the remaining ingredients and mix well. Cover and refrigerate. Keeps for 4 days.

NUTRITIONAL INFORMATION
Calories: 250 • Calories from Fat: 45
Total Fat: 5g • Saturated Fat: 0g • Dietary Fiber: 10g • Protein: 12g

Leek and Red Pepper Frittata

SERVES 2

What you will need:

1 tsp olive oil

1 leek, washed and halved lengthwise and sliced into thin moons

½ medium red bell pepper, diced

3 large eggs*

½ cup skim ricotta cheese

Salt and pepper to taste

Preheat oven broiler.

In 8-inch ovenproof skillet, heat oil over medium-high heat. Add leek and sauté until fragrant and starting to soften. Add bell peppers and continue to cook for 2 to 3 minutes.

Whisk eggs, ricotta, salt, and pepper in a medium bowl. Add egg mixture to the same skillet with the leeks. Lower heat to medium and cook, stirring constantly. When eggs start to solidify, stop stirring and use spatula to smooth out top, making sure vegetables are equally distributed. Cook over medium heat until eggs are mostly solid and bottom of frittata is golden brown.

Put skillet under broiler and cook until tip is brown and eggs are cooked through. Cut frittata into four wedges and serve.

NUTRITIONAL INFORMATION
Calories: 250 • Calories from Fat: 130
Total Fat: 15g • Saturated Fat: 6g • Dietary Fiber: 1g • Protein: 17g

Sunday Morning Apple Pancakes

SERVES 2

What you will need:

1 tbsp and 2¼ tsp whole-wheat flour

1 tbsp and 2¼ tsp unbleached all-purpose flour

2¾ tsp cornmeal

½ tsp baking powder

⅛ tsp ground ginger

⅛ tsp baking soda

⅓ cup nonfat plain yogurt

2 tbsp Eggology

2 tbsp honey

1 tbsp canola oil

⅛ apple, peeled, cored, and coarsely grated

In a blender or food processor, pulse the flours, cornmeal, baking powder, ginger, baking soda, yogurt, egg substitute, honey, and oil until just combined. By hand, stir the apples into the batter. Coat a large nonstick skillet with nonstick spray and heat over medium heat. For each pancake, spoon 2 to 3 tbsp of the batter into the skillet. Cook until lightly browned and cooked through, about 2 minutes on each side. Repeat with remaining batter.

NUTRITIONAL INFORMATION
Calories: 140 • Calories from Fat: 25
Total Fat: 3g • Saturated Fat: 0g • Dietary Fiber: 1g • Protein: 4g

Healthy Eggs Florentine

SERVES 2

What you will need:

½ cup Eggology or 2 large egg whites*

Salt and pepper to taste

½ cup thawed frozen spinach, squeezed in double layer of paper towels to remove excess liquid

1 oz low-fat goat cheese

2 slices tomato

Preheat oven to 375° F.

Lightly coat 2 1-cup ovenproof glass bowls or ceramic ramekins with cooking spray. Crack 1 egg into each ramekin and season with salt and pepper. Divide spinach evenly between 2 ramekins. Crumble goat cheese over spinach and top with tomato slice.

Place ramekins on baking sheet and bake for 15 minutes. Remove from oven. If you like your eggs well done, let them rest in ramekins for 5 minutes. Run knife around inside edges of ramekins to loosen eggs. Turn ramekins over onto plates.

Season with salt and pepper.

NUTRITIONAL INFORMATION
Calories: 120 • Calories from Fat: 60
Total Fat: 7g • Saturated Fat: 3g • Dietary Fiber: 2g • Protein: 11g

LUNCH
RECIPES

Potato, Bean, and Apple Salad

SERVES 4

What you will need:

8 oz new potatoes in their skins, scrubbed and quartered

pinch of salt

8 oz canned red kidney beans, rinsed and drained*

1 Red Delicious apple, diced and tossed in 1 tbsp lemon juice

1 small yellow bell pepper, seeded and diced

1 shallot, sliced

½ head fennel, sliced

mixed lettuce leaves

Dressing

1 tbsp red wine vinegar	1 garlic clove, crushed*
½ level tsp whole-grain mustard	2 tsp freshly chopped thyme

Place the potatoes in a saucepan and cover with water.

Bring to a boil, then add salt and simmer for 15 minutes until tender. Drain, allow to cool, and transfer into a mixing bowl. Stir in the beans, apple, pepper, shallot, and fennel.

In a separate bowl, combine all of the dressing ingredients. Pour the dressing over the salad and blend well.

Line a serving plate with the lettuce and spoon the salad on the top.

NUTRITIONAL INFORMATION
Calories: 200 • Calories from Fat: 0
Total Fat: 0g • Saturated Fat: 0g • Dietary Fiber: 13g • Protein: 11g

Buff Dad BLT (with Turkey Breast)

SERVES 1

What you will need:

1 tbsp mustard or fat-free mayonnaise

2 slices whole-grain bread

2 lettuce leaves

4 slices roasted turkey breast*

½ tomato, sliced

Spread mustard or mayonnaise evenly over bread slices. Top one slice of bread with lettuce, turkey, and tomato, then place the other slice on top. Cut in half and enjoy.

NUTRITIONAL INFORMATION
Calories: 430 • Calories from Fat: 60
Total Fat: 6g • Saturated Fat: 0.5g • Dietary Fiber: 4g • Protein: 70g

Ultimate 10-Minute Pizza

SERVES 1

What you will need:

1 whole-wheat pita

¼ cup low-fat pizza sauce

1 cooked chicken breast, sliced*

¼ red bell pepper, sliced

¼ yellow bell pepper, sliced

¼ small zucchini, sliced

¼ cup reduced-fat mozzarella cheese, shredded

Preheat oven to 425°F.

Place the pita on a baking sheet. Spoon pizza sauce evenly over the pita and top with cooked chicken, peppers, zucchini, and cheese. Bake for 10 minutes or until cheese is melted and serve.

NUTRITIONAL INFORMATION
Calories: 400 • Calories from Fat: 100
Total Fat: 11g • Saturated Fat: 4.5g • Dietary Fiber: 7g • Protein: 33g

Hearty Southwestern Chicken Salad

SERVES 4

What you will need:

¼ cup fat-free mayonnaise

¼ cup low-fat sour cream

¼ cup cilantro, chopped

1 tsp grated lime peel (zest)

1 lime, halved

½ tsp ground cumin

¼ tsp ground red pepper

4 cooked chicken breasts, cut into bite-size pieces*

1 can (15 oz) black beans, drained and rinsed*

1 red bell pepper, diced

½ red onion, chopped

2 heads Bibb lettuce, separated into leaves

In a large mixing bowl, combine mayonnaise, sour cream, cilantro, lime zest, juice from lime halves, cumin, and ground red pepper. Then stir in chicken, beans, bell pepper, and onion.

Divide lettuce evenly among four plates and top with chicken salad.

NUTRITIONAL INFORMATION
Calories: 220 • Calories from Fat: 40
Total Fat: 4g • Saturated Fat: 2g • Dietary Fiber: 9g • Protein: 19g

Fruit and Nut Chicken Salad

SERVES 2

What you will need:

2 cooked chicken breasts, chopped*

½ cup seedless red grapes, chilled and halved

½ cup green grapes, chilled and halved

1 apple, cored and diced

½ cup fat-free mayonnaise

1 lemon, halved

¼ tsp ground black pepper

2 cups baby romaine leaves

2 tbsp chopped pecans

In a mixing bowl, combine cooked chicken, red and green grapes, apple, mayonnaise, juice from lemon halves, and black pepper. Place the baby romaine leaves on two plates and spoon chicken mixture over lettuce.

Sprinkle with chopped pecans and enjoy.

NUTRITIONAL INFORMATION
Calories: 440 • Calories from Fat: 150
Total Fat: 16g • Saturated Fat: 3.5g • Dietary Fiber: 7g • Protein: 36g

---

T-Booster Beef Sub

SERVES 1

What you will need:

1 whole-grain roll

1 tbsp fat-free mayonnaise

2 lettuce leaves

½ tomato, sliced

4 slices of lean roast beef, sliced*

1 slice of red onion

Slice roll horizontally in half and spread with fat-free mayonnaise. Top with lettuce leaves, tomato slices, roast beef, and onion. Serve and enjoy.

NUTRITIONAL INFORMATION
Calories: 360 • Calories from Fat: 70
Total Fat: 7g • Saturated Fat: 2g • Dietary Fiber: 9g • Protein: 22g

SNACK
RECIPES

Blueberry Protein Blast

SERVES 1

What you will need:

½ cup low-fat cottage cheese*

6 oz light fat-free blueberry yogurt

Combine cottage cheese and blueberry yogurt in a bowl. Serve and enjoy.

NUTRITIONAL INFORMATION
Calories: 180 • Calories from Fat: 15
Total Fat: 1.5g • Saturated Fat: 1g • Dietary Fiber: 0g • Protein: 20g

Apple and Cheese Quickie

SERVES 1

What you will need:

1 apple

1 part-skim string cheese

Place apple and cheese on a plate. Enjoy.

NUTRITIONAL INFORMATION
Calories: 160 • Calories from Fat: 50
Total Fat: 6g • Saturated Fat: 3.5g • Dietary Fiber: 5g • Protein: 8g

Low-Fat Tuna Melt

SERVES 1

What you will need:

3 oz canned tuna, packed in water

5 whole-wheat crackers

1 tbsp low-fat cheddar cheese

Spread tuna on whole-wheat crackers. Sprinkle cheese and microwave for 10 seconds.

NUTRITIONAL INFORMATION
Calories: 290 • Calories from Fat: 70
Total Fat: 8g • Saturated Fat: 2g • Dietary Fiber: 4g • Protein: 27g

Raspberry Hunger-Cruncher

SERVES 1

What you will need:

2 tbsp balsamic vinegar

1 cup raspberries

1 packet sugar substitute

1 cup fat-free yogurt

8 chopped walnuts

In a bowl, pour vinegar over berries and marinate for 10 minutes. Mix sweetener and yogurt until well blended. Spoon berries over yogurt and sprinkle with walnuts.

NUTRITIONAL INFORMATION
Calories: 290 • Calories from Fat: 100
Total Fat: 11g • Saturated Fat: 1g • Dietary Fiber: 1g • Protein: 12g

Turkey Roll-ups

SERVES 1

What you will need:

   2 lean turkey slices*

   2 slices low-fat Swiss cheese

   4 whole-wheat crackers

Place one turkey slice over one slice of Swiss cheese. Roll up together and eat. Repeat with second turkey slice and cheese. Finish snack with whole-wheat crackers.

NUTRITIONAL INFORMATION
Calories: 270 • Calories from Fat: 70
Total Fat: 8g • Saturated Fat: 2g • Dietary Fiber: 3g • Protein: 22g

DINNER
RECIPES

Beef Burritos

SERVES 4

What you will need:

1 lb lean ground beef*

1 tbsp olive oil

½ cup water

1 packet Old El Paso taco seasoning

4 whole-wheat tortillas

1 cup diced tomato

1 cup shredded lettuce

¼ cup diced red onion

4 oz shredded low-fat cheddar cheese or soy cheese

low-fat sour cream (optional)

hot sauce (optional)

Sauté the ground beef in oil with the water until beef is brown. Add the seasoning and let simmer until the water has evaporated off.

Fill the tortillas with the cooked ground beef. Add the tomato, lettuce, onion, and cheese. If desired, add hot sauce and sour cream. Fold and enjoy.

NUTRITIONAL INFORMATION
Calories: 380 • Calories from Fat: 120
Total Fat: 13g • Saturated Fat: 3.5g • Dietary Fiber: 3g • Protein: 33g

Chicken Vegetable Pizza

SERVES 6

What you will need:

1 fat-free deep-dish pizza crust

2 tbsp fat-free chicken broth

1 lb fat-free chicken tenders*

1 tsp garlic powder*

1½ tsp onion powder

2 tsp dried basil

2 cups fat-free pizza sauce

2 cups fat-free shredded mozzarella cheese

1 medium yellow bell pepper, sliced thin

1 medium red bell pepper, sliced thin

1 cup sliced mushrooms

1 medium red onion, sliced thin

⅓ cup fat-free Parmesan cheese

Preheat oven to 425° F.

Lightly spray the deep-dish pizza pan with nonfat cooking spray. Press pizza crust into pan. Prick several times with a fork and bake in preheated oven 10–12 minutes until lightly browned.

Lightly spray large nonstick skillet with nonfat cooking spray. Pour chicken broth into skillet and heat over medium-high heat until simmering.

Add the chicken tenders to the broth and sprinkle with garlic powder, onion powder, and basil. Cook over medium heat, stirring frequently, for 8–10 minutes until chicken is no longer pink. Using a slotted spoon, remove the chicken from the skillet and cut into bite-sized pieces.

Pour pizza sauce over crust. Sprinkle half the mozzarella cheese over sauce. Top with chicken, yellow and red peppers, mushrooms, and sliced onion. Sprinkle with remaining mozzarella cheese and Parmesan cheese.

Bake in preheated oven 10–12 minutes until cheese is completely melted.

NUTRITIONAL INFORMATION
Calories: 320 • Calories from Fat: 45
Total Fat: 5g • Saturated Fat: 1.5g • Dietary Fiber: 3g • Protein: 43g

---

Beef and Bean Chili

SERVES 6

What you will need:

2 cups uncooked brown rice

2 lbs lean beef stew meat (trimmed of fat), cut in 1-inch cubes*

3 tbsp vegetable oil

2 cups water

2 tsp minced garlic*

1 large onion, finely chopped

1 tbsp flour

2 tsp chili powder

1 green pepper, chopped

2 lbs tomatoes, chopped (approximately 3 cups)

1 tbsp oregano

1 tsp cumin

2 cups canned kidney beans, drained and rinsed*

Prepare rice according to package directions. Sauté the meat in a large skillet with half of the vegetable oil. Once brown, add the water and simmer, covered, for 1 hour, until meat is tender.

Heat the remaining vegetable oil in a second skillet. Add garlic and onion and cook over low heat until onion is softened. Add the flour and cook 2 minutes.

Pour the garlic-onion-flour mixture into the cooked meat and then add the remaining ingredients to the meat mixture. Stir and simmer for 30 minutes. Serve over rice.

NUTRITIONAL INFORMATION
Calories: 410 • Calories from Fat: 150
Total Fat: 17g • Saturated Fat: 4g • Dietary Fiber: 7g • Protein: 41g

Grilled Chicken Kabobs

SERVES 4

What you will need:

1 cup uncooked brown rice

4 chicken breasts cut into 1½-inch squares*

2 green bell peppers, cut into 1½-inch pieces

2 red bell peppers, cut into 1½-inch pieces

12 fresh mushrooms, whole

1 onion, cut into wedges

1 tbsp olive oil

2 tsp chicken seasoning

Prepare rice according to package directions and preheat grill.

On four skewers, alternately thread a piece of chicken, green pepper, red pepper, mushroom, and onion. Repeat until all ingredients are used. Then lightly brush the kabobs with olive oil and sprinkle with seasoning.

Grill kabobs for 5 minutes, then turn and grill for another 5 minutes. Serve with rice.

NUTRITIONAL INFORMATION
Calories: 380 • Calories from Fat: 60
Total Fat: 7g • Saturated Fat: 1g • Dietary Fiber: 5g • Protein: 33g

Low-Fat Tangy BBQ Chicken

SERVES 2

What you will need:

½ cup uncooked brown rice	hot pepper sauce, to taste
3 tsp olive oil	2 cloves garlic, minced*
2 chicken breasts*	¼ tsp ground black pepper
½ onion, diced	1 tsp Worcestershire sauce
1 cup tomato juice	½ red bell pepper, diced
⅓ cup white vinegar	1 tbsp chives, sliced

Prepare brown rice according to package. While the rice is cooking, heat 2 teaspoons of olive oil in a skillet over medium heat. Add chicken breast, cover, and cook chicken for 6 minutes. Turn breasts over and cook for another 6 minutes until they are no longer pink in the center.

Heat the remaining olive oil in a medium saucepan over medium heat. Add onion and sauté until golden brown. Add tomato juice, vinegar, hot pepper sauce, garlic, black pepper, and Worcestershire sauce. Stir well and simmer over low heat for 10 minutes.

When chicken is done, add it to sauce and simmer for another 3 minutes. Stir the diced bell pepper and chives into the cooked rice. Serve rice with chicken.

NUTRITIONAL INFORMATION
Calories: 260 • Calories from Fat: 80
Total Fat: 9g • Saturated Fat: 2g • Dietary Fiber: 2g • Protein: 20g

Hearty Beef Stew

SERVES 4

What you will need:

1 onion, chopped

1 lb of round steak, cut into 1-inch chunks*

2½ cups low-fat, reduced-sodium beef broth

4 medium-sized potatoes, peeled and cut into 1-inch chunks

1 lb baby carrots, sliced

2 celery stalks, sliced

¼ cup tomato paste

½ tsp ground black pepper

2 tbsp Worcestershire sauce

1 bay leaf

¼ cup red wine (optional)

2 tbsp fresh parsley, chopped

Lightly coat a large pot with cooking spray and place on medium-high heat. Add onions and sauté until tender. Then add beef chunks and sauté. Once brown on all sides, add beef broth, potato chunks, carrots, celery, tomato paste, black pepper, Worcestershire sauce, bay leaf, and red wine, and bring to a boil. Reduce heat and simmer for 90 minutes or until meat is tender.

Remove bay leaf and spoon beef stew into four bowls. Sprinkle with parsley.

NUTRITIONAL INFORMATION
Calories: 360 • Calories from Fat: 40
Total Fat: 4.5g • Saturated Fat: 1.5g • Dietary Fiber: 6g • Protein: 34g

Make-Ahead Garlic Yogurt Sirloin

SERVES 2

What you will need:

½ cup low-fat plain yogurt

¼ cup chopped fresh parsley

1 tbsp lemon juice

½ tbsp paprika

1 clove garlic, minced*

1 pinch salt

2 (4-ounce) sirloin steaks*

⅛ cup low-fat mayonnaise

Combine all ingredients except steak and mayonnaise in a bowl; mix well. Divide mixture in half. Combine half the mixture and steaks in a food-safe plastic bag. Turn to coat. Marinate overnight in refrigerator. Add mayo to remaining mix; refrigerate.

Place steaks on grill heated to high, turning once, until internal temperature is 155° F. Serve topped with leftover marinade.

NUTRITIONAL INFORMATION
Calories: 220 • Calories from Fat: 70
Total Fat: 7g • Saturated Fat: 2.5g • Dietary Fiber: 1g • Protein: 29g

Mama Mia Chicken Parmesan

SERVES 2

What you will need:

2 egg whites*

⅓ cup Italian seasoned bread crumbs

4 tbsp reduced-fat Parmesan cheese, grated and divided

2 chicken breasts*

4 oz uncooked spinach pasta

1 cup low-fat pasta sauce

2 cups baby spinach leaves

Preheat oven to 400° F.

In a mixing bowl, beat egg whites with a fork until slightly frothy. Then mix bread crumbs and 2 tablespoons of Parmesan cheese in a pie plate. Dip chicken in the egg whites and then into the bread crumb mixture, coating both sides.

Lightly coat a baking sheet with cooking spray. Place chicken breasts on the baking sheet and bake for approximately 12 minutes. Turn over and cook for another 12 minutes or until chicken is no longer pink in the center.

While the chicken is baking, prepare spinach pasta according to package directions. Warm pasta in a saucepan if necessary.

Divide spinach leaves between two plates. Layer spinach pasta and chicken breasts over leaves and top with pasta sauce and remaining Parmesan cheese.

NUTRITIONAL INFORMATION
Calories: 410 • Calories from Fat: 100
Total Fat: 11g • Saturated Fat: 2g • Dietary Fiber: 5g • Protein: 39g

Savory Grilled Fish Tacos

SERVES 4

What you will need:

1 tbsp olive oil

4 limes, halved

5 cloves garlic, minced*

2 tsp ground cumin

1½ lbs swordfish or tuna

1 ripe avocado, peeled, pitted, and diced

¼ red onion, minced

2 jalapeños, seeded and minced

2 tbsp fresh cilantro, chopped

8 6-inch whole-wheat flour tortillas

8 lettuce leaves

Preheat grill to medium.

Combine olive oil, juice of 3 limes, 4 garlic cloves, and 1 teaspoon cumin in a shallow bowl or pie plate. Then add fish to this marinade and let it soak up the flavors for 15 minutes at room temperature, turning once. While fish is marinating, in a separate bowl stir together the remaining lime juice, garlic, and cumin with diced avocado, onion, jalapeños, and cilantro.

Place the marinated fish on the hot grill and cook for 5 minutes. Turn over and cook for an additional 5 minutes. Place fish on cutting board and cut into thin strips.

While grill is still hot, place tortillas directly on it and grill them for 30 seconds each side. Place two tortillas on each plate. Put a lettuce leaf in each tortilla, filled with a portion of grilled, sliced fish and top with avocado salsa. Fold tortillas over and enjoy.

NUTRITIONAL INFORMATION
Calories: 600 • Calories from Fat: 170
Total Fat: 19g • Saturated Fat: 2g • Dietary Fiber: 10g • Protein: 48g

Pasta Lovers
Spaghetti and Meatballs

SERVES 6

What you will need:

1½ lbs of lean ground turkey or ground beef*

2 egg whites*

½ cup dry bread crumbs

¼ cup water

½ onion, finely chopped

2 cloves garlic, minced

¼ cup fresh parsley, minced*

2 tsp dried basil

1 tsp ground black pepper

3 cups low-fat marinara pasta sauce

12 oz uncooked spaghetti

¼ cup reduced-fat Parmesan cheese

Preheat oven broiler.

In a bowl, combine turkey or beef, egg whites, bread crumbs, water, onion, garlic, parsley, basil, and black pepper. Mix ingredients together and then shape into 1½-inch meatballs. Arrange the balls on a baking sheet and place under broiler for 10–12 minutes, turning occasionally until they are browned on all sides.

In a large saucepan, combine pasta sauce and cooked meatballs. Simmer over low heat for about 20 minutes. While the meatballs are cooking in the sauce, prepare the pasta as per the package directions.

Place a serving of spaghetti on each plate, spoon over sauce and meatballs, and enjoy.

NUTRITIONAL INFORMATION
Calories: 510 • Calories from Fat: 90
Total Fat: 9g • Saturated Fat: 2g • Dietary Fiber: 2g • Protein: 34g

Five-Minute Mediterranean Salmon

SERVES 2

What you will need:

1 tbsp extra-virgin olive oil

1 clove garlic, chopped*

1 cup chopped tomatoes

¼ cup chopped basil

2 tbsp pine nuts

2 salmon steaks (approximately ½ lb each)

2 cups steamed broccoli*

1 cup fingerling potatoes, cooked until tender

Fill a saucepan full of water and bring to a boil.

While waiting for the water to boil, sauté garlic in olive oil in a nonstick pan until tender. Add chopped tomatoes, basil, and pine nuts to the garlic. Simmer together in the nonstick pan until heated thoroughly.

Add salmon to boiling water and poach until done (about 5 minutes). Remove from water and place on a dish. Spoon tomato garlic mixture over salmon. Serve with broccoli and fingerling potatoes.

NUTRITIONAL INFORMATION
Calories: 490 • Calories from Fat: 240
Total Fat: 27g • Saturated Fat: 4.5g • Dietary Fiber: 4g • Protein: 53g

Spicy Beef Stir-Fry

SERVES 2

What you will need:

1 tbsp olive oil

1 onion, sliced

1 clove garlic, chopped*

1 lb lean sirloin steak, cut into strips*

½ red bell pepper, sliced

½ green bell pepper, sliced

1 jalapeño, sliced

1 cup brown rice, cooked

In a nonstick pan over medium heat, add olive oil and cook onion and garlic until tender. Add steak and peppers and continue to cook until steak is done. Serve with brown rice.

NUTRITIONAL INFORMATION
Calories: 630 • Calories from Fat: 190
Total Fat: 22g • Saturated Fat: 6g • Dietary Fiber: 5g • Protein: 71g

DESSERTS

Chewy Chocolate Brownies

SERVES 12

What you will need:

½ cup soy flour

¼ cup whole-wheat flour

½ cup Splenda granular

¼ cup unsweetened cocoa
  powder

½ tsp baking powder

¼ tsp salt

¼ cup canola oil

2 tsp vanilla extract

6 egg whites, beaten*

¼ cup unsweetened applesauce

¼ cup water

⅓ cup walnut pieces

Preheat oven to 350° F and lightly coat an 8" x 8" square baking dish with butter-flavored cooking spray.

In a bowl, sift together soy flour, whole-wheat flour, Splenda, cocoa powder, baking powder, and salt. In another bowl, combine canola oil, vanilla extract, egg whites, applesauce, and water. Pour liquid mixture into flour mixture and stir just until combined. Mixture may be lumpy.

Pour brownie batter into baking dish and sprinkle with walnuts. Bake for 15 minutes or until edges spring back when touched gently. The center of the brownies will be soft.

Serve one brownie with a glass of your favorite protein powder mixed with water or skim milk.

NUTRITIONAL INFORMATION
Calories: 110 • Calories from Fat: 60
Total Fat: 7g • Saturated Fat: 0.5g • Dietary Fiber: 2g • Protein: 5g

Craving-Buster Sundae

SERVES 2

What you will need:

½ cup skim milk

1 scoop (about 24g of protein) vanilla protein powder (whey or soy)

2 cups frozen banana slices (2 medium bananas)

4 tsp chocolate syrup

4 tbsp fat-free Cool Whip

2 tsp chopped nuts

2 maraschino cherries

Pour skim milk into blender and add protein powder. Blend on high speed for about 15 seconds. Add frozen banana slices and blend on high speed for 45 seconds or until smooth.

Spoon into two dessert bowls and top each with 2 teaspoons of chocolate syrup, 2 tablespoons of Cool Whip, a teaspoon of chopped nuts, and a maraschino cherry.

NUTRITIONAL INFORMATION
Calories: 270 • Calories from Fat: 30
Total Fat: 3.5g • Saturated Fat: 0.5g • Dietary Fiber: 3g • Protein: 13g

Appendix: *Buff Dad* Meal Plan Forms

	DAY 1	DAY 2	DAY 3
WEEK _____			
BREAKFAST			
Snack			
LUNCH			
Snack			
DINNER			
Snack			

DAY 4	DAY 5	DAY 6	DAY 7

Week 1 Sample

	DAY 1	DAY 2	DAY 3
BREAKFAST	Protein Power Pancakes	*Buff Dad* Breakfast Turk-wich	Early-Bird Pizza
Snack	Blueberry Protein Blast	Low-Fat Tuna Melt	2 oz low-fat cheese or 2 string cheese
LUNCH	Ultimate 10-Minute Pizza	*Buff Dad* BLT with Turkey	T-Booster Beef Sub
Snack	1 banana (small)	½ cup 1% cottage cheese 10 almonds	Blueberry Protein Blast
DINNER	Beef Burritos	Chicken Vegetable Pizza	Grilled Chicken Kabobs
Snack	Chewy Chocolate Brownies	Craving-Buster Sundae	1 plum or other small fruit

DAY 4	DAY 5	DAY 6	DAY 7
Strawberry-Banana Power Shake	Mexican Egg Burrito	Make-Ahead Oatmeal	Sunday Morning Apple Pancakes
Apple and Cheese Quickie	Turkey Roll-Ups	Raspberry Hunger-Cruncher	Blueberry Protein Blast
Potato, Bean, and Apple Salad	Hearty Southwestern Chicken Salad	*Buff Dad* BLT with Turkey	Ultimate 10-Minute Pizza
1 small apple 1 tbsp all-natural peanut butter	1 cup pineapple	½ cup 1% cottage cheese 10 almonds	Apple and Cheese Quickie
Beef and Bean Chili	Low-Fat Tangy BBQ Chicken	Hearty Beef Stew	Make-Ahead Garlic Yogurt Sirloin
Chewy Chocolate Brownies	1 cup low-fat yogurt (60 cals or less) 10 peanuts	Craving-Buster Sundae	1 cup low-fat yogurt (60 cals or less)

Week 2 Sample

	DAY 1	DAY 2	DAY 3
BREAKFAST	Healthy Eggs Florentine	Protein Power Pancakes	Mexican Egg Burrito
Snack	1 low-fat yogurt (60 cals or less) 10 almonds	1 small apple 1 tbsp all-natural peanut butter	Blueberry Protein Blast
LUNCH	*Buff Dad* BLT with Turkey	Potato, Bean, and Apple Salad	T-Booster Beef Sub
Snack	Blueberry Protein Blast	Apple and Cheese Quickie	Turkey Roll-ups
DINNER	Mama Mia Chicken Parmesan	Savory Grilled Fish Tacos	Pasta Lovers Spaghetti and Meatballs
Snack	1 low-fat chocolate pudding	Chewy Chocolate Brownies	2 cups watermelon

DAY 4	DAY 5	DAY 6	DAY 7
Strawberry-Banana Power Shake	*Buff Dad* Breakfast Turk-wich	Early-Bird Pizza	Leek and Red Pepper Frittata
1 low-fat yogurt (60 cals or less) 10 almonds	Apple and Cheese Quickie	Raspberry Hunger-Cruncher	Turkey Roll-Ups
Ultimate 10-Minute Pizza	Chicken Pita Sandwich: • 4 oz chicken breast baked, broiled, or grilled • 1 whole-wheat pita • 5 leaves romaine • 1 tsp Dijon mustard	*Buff Dad* BLT with Turkey	Fruit and Nut Chicken Salad
1 apple 1 tbsp all-natural peanut butter	Low-Fat Tuna Melt	Blueberry Protein Blast	1 kiwi or small fruit 2 oz low-fat cheese
Spicy Beef Stir-Fry	Five-Minute Mediterranean Salmon	Beef and Bean Chili	Grilled Chicken Kabobs
Craving-Buster Sundae	1 low-fat yogurt (60 cals or less) 10 almonds	1 low-fat chocolate pudding	Chewy Chocolate Brownies

Week 3 Sample

	DAY 1	DAY 2	DAY 3
BREAKFAST	Strawberry-Banana Power Shake	Healthy Eggs Florentine	Early-Bird Pizza
Snack	1 cup fresh strawberries	1 small apple 1 tbsp all-natural peanut butter	Blueberry Protein Blast
LUNCH	Hearty Southwestern Chicken Salad	Ultimate 10-Minute Pizza	Potato, Bean, and Apple Salad
Snack	1 banana (small)	Blueberry Protein Blast	Turkey Roll-Ups
DINNER	Hearty Beef Stew	Low-Fat Tangy BBQ Chicken	Make-Ahead Garlic Yogurt Sirloin
Snack	Chewy Chocolate Brownies	Craving-Buster Sundae	1 plum or other small fruit

DAY 4	DAY 5	DAY 6	DAY 7
Make-Ahead Oatmeal	Protein Power Pancakes	Mexican Egg Burrito	Sunday Morning Apple Pancakes
1 low-fat yogurt (60 cals or less) 10 almonds	Apple and Cheese Quickie	Turkey Roll-ups	Low-Fat Tuna Melt
Buff Dad BLT with Turkey	T-Booster Beef Sub	Hearty Southwestern Chicken Salad	Ultimate 10-Minute Pizza
1 small apple 1 tbsp all-natural peanut butter	Raspberry Hunger-Cruncher	Apple and Cheese Quickie	Turkey Roll-ups
Savory Grilled Fish Tacos	Mama Mia Chicken Parmesan	Pasta Lovers Spaghetti and Meatballs	Beef Burritos
Blueberry Protein Blast	1 low-fat yogurt (60 cals or less) 10 peanuts	1 peach or any small fruit	1 cup low-fat yogurt (60 cals or less)

Week 4 Sample

	DAY 1	DAY 2	DAY 3
BREAKFAST	Strawberry-Banana Power Shake	Early-Bird Pizza	Healthy Eggs Florentine
Snack	1 low-fat yogurt (60 cals or less) 10 almonds	1 small apple 1 tbsp all-natural peanut butter	Turkey Roll-Up
LUNCH	*Buff Dad* BLT with Turkey	Hearty Southwestern Chicken Salad	Ultimate 10-Minute Pizza
Snack	1 apple	Blueberry Protein Blast	Apple and Cheese Quickie
DINNER	Spicy Beef Stir-Fry	Grilled Chicken Kabobs	Chicken and Vegetable Pizza
Snack	1 low-fat chocolate pudding	Chewy Chocolate Brownies	Craving-Buster Sundae

DAY 4	DAY 5	DAY 6	DAY 7
Protein Power Pancakes	Mexican Egg Burrito	*Buff Dad* Breakfast Turk-wich	Sunday Morning Apple Pancakes
Blueberry Protein Blast	1 small apple 1 tbsp all-natural peanut butter	Raspberry Hunger-Cruncher	Low-Fat Tuna Melt
Potato, Bean, and Apple Salad	T-Booster Beef Sub	*Buff Dad* BLT with Turkey	Fruit and Nut Chicken Salad
2 tbsp all-natural peanut butter 1 apple	1 banana	Turkey Roll-Up	Raspberry Hunger-Cruncher
Beef Burritos	Savory Grilled Fish Tacos	Hearty Beef Stew	Mama Mia Chicken Parmesan
1 banana	1 low-fat yogurt (60 cals or less) 10 almonds	1 low-fat chocolate pudding	Chewy Chocolate Brownies

EGGOLOGY

More protein and less fat

One of the keys to the *Buff Dad* dietary plan is to ensure you have enough protein in your diet so that your body never needs to take it from your muscles. While lean beef, chicken and fish are a good way to get this protein, a fast and simple way to start your day is with egg whites such those found in Eggology.

Eggology contains no fat, no cholesterol and carbohydrates. What you are getting is 100 percent protein along with great taste. One of the best things about Eggology is that it's pure egg whites, which is great for buff dads like us. Unlike fish, chicken turkey, and other protein powders that have to be broken down by the body before being used, egg whites are absorbed instantly. But what makes Eggology different from other products is that it's the only one that acts exactly like regular egg whites. In fact, you can whip them into meringue if you really wanted to.

Eggology egg whites are versatile, making them a perfect addition to the buff dad day. They are safe to drink raw in a shake or smoothie or can be made into omelets, egg sandwiches, and quiches—all without adding extra fat or cholesterol to your diet. Whip them for breakfast or simply microwave them anytime for a high protein snack.

I don't know about you, but carrying real eggs around in my briefcase just never seemed logical. Eggology comes in single serving containers so you can take them anywhere. Less than two minutes in the microwave and you have instant protein to roll up in tortilla, spoon onto whole wheat crackers or eat on the way to the gym—plus with a whooping 7 grams of protein and only 30 calories per serving, you can't go wrong.

Perfecto Tex-Mex Frittata

SERVING SIZE: 2

What you will need:

⅓ cup thinly sliced green onions

3 tablespoons canned chopped green chilies

1 teaspoon chili powder

½ teaspoon ground cumin

6 ounces *Eggology* fresh egg whites, lightly beaten

1 (15-ounce) can no salt-added black beans, rinsed and drained

   cooking spray

3 garlic cloves, minced

½ cup (2 ounces) shredded Monterey jack cheese with jalapeno peppers

2 tablespoons fat-free sour cream

2 tablespoons salsa

1 tablespoon chopped fresh cilantro

1. Preheat oven to 450°F.

2. Combine first 6 ingredients in a bowl; stir well. Set aside.

3. Coat a 10-inch nonstick skillet with cooking spray; place over medium heat until hot. Add garlic; sauté 1 minute. Stir in bean mixture; spread evenly in bottom of skillet. Cook over medium-low heat 5 minutes or until almost set.

4. Wrap handle of skillet with foil; place skillet in oven, and bake at 450 degrees for 5 minutes or until set. Sprinkle with cheese; bake an additional minute or until cheese melts. Top each serving with sour cream and salsa; sprinkle with cilantro.

For more recipe ideas or information, go to www.eggology.com.

REFERENCES

Badman, M. Low-carb diet finding: Study identifies new regulator of fat metabolism. *Science Daily,* June 6, 2007.

Bergman, BC, GA Brooks. Respiratory gas-exchange ratios during graded exercise in fed and fasted trained and untrained men. *Journal of Applied Physiology,* 1999, 86:2.

Bhasin, S, L Woodhouse, R Casaburi, AB Singh, R Phong Mac, M Lee, K Yarasheski, I Sinha-Hikim, C Dzekov, J Dzekov, L Magliano, and TW Storer. Older men are as responsive as young men to the anabolic effects of graded doses of testosterone on the skeletal muscle. *The Journal of Clinical Endocrinology & Metabolism,* Vol. 90, No. 2, 678–688, 2005.

Bosco, C, R Colli, R Bonomi, S P Von Duvillard, and A Viru. "Monitoring strength training: neuromuscular and hormonal profile." Department of Physical Medicine and Rehabilitation, Faculty of Medicine and Surgery, University of Rome Tor Vergata, Rome, Italy; Department of Biology of Physical Activity, University of Jyvaskyla, Finland; Human Performance, Department of HPER, University of North Dakota, ND; and Institute of Exercise Biology, University of Tartu, Estonia. March 1988.

Brehm, BA. Recovery energy expenditure for steady state exercise in runners and non-exercisers. *Medicine and Science in Sports and Exercise,* 1986, 18:205.

Brybner, BW. The effects of exercise intensity on body composition, weight loss and dietary composition in women. *Journal of American College of Nutrition,* 1997, 16:68–73.

Collins, P. Testosterone and the cardiovascular system—friend or foe? National Heart & Lung Institute, Imperial College of Science, Technology and Medicine, London, Men's Health Forum, December 2001.

Conniff, R. Testosterone under attack. *Men's Health,* September 2007.

Cooper, B. Are you doing too much cardio? *Men's Fitness,* October 2004.

Cressey, E. The MF testosterone program. *Men's Fitness,* May 2007.

Freedman, DS, TR O'Brien, WD Flanders, F DeStefano, and JJ Barboriak. Relation of serum testosterone levels to high density lipoprotein cholesterol and other characteristics in men. *Arteriosclerosis and Thrombosis,* Vol. 11, 307–315, 1991.

Giorgi, A, RP Weatherby, and PW Murphy. Muscular strength, body composition and health responses to the use of testosterone enanthate: a double blind study. School of Exercise Science and Sports Management, Southern Cross University, Lismore, NSW, Australia, 1999.

King, BJ. *The Awaken Your Body Plan.* Transforming Health Inc., 2007.

Krucoff, C. Working out with kids. Foodfit.com, February 2005.

Loebel, CC, and WJ Kraemer. A brief review: testosterone and resistance training in men. *Journal of Strength and Conditioning,* 1998, 12(1).

McCarty, MF. Optimizing exercise for fat loss. *Medical Hypothesis,* 1995, 44:325–30.

Ostbye, T, L Bastian, H Weng, D Taylor, and B Moser. Parental obesity; number of children linked to obesity for mom and dad. Duke University Medical Center, 2004.

Pasternak, H. *5-Factor Fitness.* New York: GP Putnam and Sons, 2004.

Phillips, B. *Body for Life: 12 Weeks to Mental and Physical Strength.* HarperCollins Publishers, 2002.

Schuler, L. *The Men's Health Home Workout Bible.* Rodale, 2001.

Schuler, L. *The Testosterone Advantage Plan.* Fireside, 2003.

Bhasin, S, TW Storer, N Asbel-Sethi, A Kilbourne, R Hays, I Sinha-Hikim, R Shen, S Arver, and G Beall. Effects of testosterone replacement with a nongenital, transdermal system, androderm, in human immunodeficiency virus-infected men with low testosterone levels. *The Journal of Clinical Endocrinology & Metabolism*, Vol. 83, No. 9, 3155–3162, 1998.

Swan, Shanna, EP Elkin, and L Fenster. Have sperm densities declined? A reanalysis of global trend data. *Environmental Health Perspectives* 105(11):1228–1232, 1997.

Teegarden, SL and TL Bale. Decreases in dietary preference produce increased emotionality and risk for dietary relapse, *Biological Psychiatry*, Vol. 61, Issue 9, May 1, 2007.

Thibaudeau, C. Testosterone training. Trulyhuge.com, March 2007.

Travison, TG, AB Araujo, AB O'Donnell, V Kupelian, and JB McKinlay. A population-level decline in serum testosterone levels in American men. *Journal of Clinical Endocrinology and Metabolism*, 92:196–202, 2007.

Urban RJ, YH Bodenburg, C Gilkison, J Foxworth, AR Coggan, RR Wolfe, and A Ferrando. Testosterone administration to elderly men increases skeletal muscle strength and protein synthesis. *American Journal of Physiology* 269: E820–E826, 1995.

Venuto, T. *Burn the Fat, Feed the Muscle.* Fitness Renaissance, 2007.

Volek, J, W Kraemer, J Bush, T Incledon, and M Boetes. Testosterone and cortisol in relationship to dietary nutrients and resistance exercise. Center for Sports Medicine, Department of Kinesiology, Noll Physiological Research Center, and Center for Cell Research. *Journal of Applied Physiology*, Vol. 82, No. 1, 49–54, January 1997.

Willcutts, KF, AR Wilson, and KK Grunewald. Energy metabolism during exercise at different time intervals following a meal. *International Journal of Sports Medicine*, 9:240–243, 1988.

Winters, J. Streamline your workout and other tricks on how to fit fitness into your life. Dadmag.com, February 2005.

Zava, David. Testosterone levels declining in men at younger ages: hormone tests reflect global trend, ZRT Laboratories, August 2007.

INDEX

Page numbers followed by an f or p indicate figures or photographs.